The Periodontal Solution:
Healthy Gums Naturally

D1239442

The Periodontal Solution: Healthy Gums Naturally

A Guide to Saving Your Teeth,
Your Money
and Your Health

By James Harrison, D.D.S., F.A.G.D., F.I.A.O.M.T.
with Constance Clark

The Periodontal Solution: Healthy Gums Naturally

by James Harrison, D.D.S.
with Constance Clark

Corinthian Health Press
1730 Federal Highway, Suite 206
Delray Beach, FL 33483
561/704-0038

Find us on the World Wide Web at:
http://www.theintegrativedentist.com

Cover design: Chris Heller
Interior design and production: Terri Shafer (writtenedge.com)
Illustrations: Billy Schwartz

Disclaimer
This book is intended as an educational tool to acquaint the reader with alternative methods of preventing and treating gum disease. Every effort has been made to make this book as complete and accurate as possible. The author and publisher shall have neither liability nor any responsibility to any person or entity with respect to any loss, damage or injury caused or alleged to be caused directly or indirectly by the information contained in this book. The information presented herein is in no way intended as a substitute for dental or medical counseling.

Copyright

Trademarks

ISBN 0-9716553-0-8

Printed and bound in the United States of America

Dedicated

To my father, Dan Harrison, a man of quiet wisdom. His depth of knowledge always provided more than a simple answer, teaching me the complexities of life.

To my mother, Marilyn Harrison. It has been a great comfort to know you are always there for me.

To my daughter, Nina, a gifted young woman who is a continual source of joy.

Table of Contents

Acknowledgements

I would like to express my gratitude to my patients for their abundant questions and challenging answers; to my friends and colleagues in the IAOMT for the clues to the puzzles; to the masters whose groundbreaking work sparked new ideas.

I want to especially thank Frank D'Amelio, Sr., a visionary in the herbal industry for encouraging us to write this book and inspiring the development of these new products. I am also grateful for the assistance of my dental staff, who were instrumental in running the research project: Mary Scorsone, Karri Valot-Homer, Ann Bent, Deborah Farmer and Jenny Avery.

Thank you, Terri Shafer, of Written Edge for helping to organize and transform this manuscript into a book. Thank you, Billy Schwartz, a talented artist, for transforming thoughts into pictures. Thank you, Chris Heller, for the book cover and layout. And thank you, Charles Owens, for help in transforming the video images of microbes into digital form.

To all of our friends and family who have given time and constructive suggestions, we are grateful.

The Journey

For over twenty years, I have been dedicated to the practice of what I call Integrative Dentistry. Integrative Dentistry combines science-based, high quality dentistry with holistic principles. From the beginning, my integrative approach was a success. However, I was concerned with many patients failure to respond to conventional treatment for gum or periodontal disease. After becoming increasingly frustrated with the prescribed approach of pocket cleaning and surgery, I began investigating this major dental challenge.

As the old proverb says, the journey of a thousand miles begins with one step. A colleague and nutritional consultant, Lino Stanchich, suggested that I study with Melvin Page, a biochemist and periodontist. Dr. Page had written several books on blood chemistry and the health effects on the body. Through looking primarily at the calcium to phosphorus ratio, he demonstrated that balanced body chemistry was essential to healthy gums. I contacted Dr. Page, studied with him, and so the journey began.

I am particularly proud to be a fellow of the International Academy of Oral Medicine and Toxicology (iaomt.org), a group of dentists, physicians and researchers from around the world. Their mission is to promote the health of the public by compiling scientific research relating to the biocompatibility of oral/dental materials.

My continued investigation led me to the research of Dr. Paul Keyes, whose work focused on controlling bacteria in the mouth. At his suggestion, I purchased a phase-contrast microscope to examine the plaque that forms on teeth. (This kind of microscope allows the viewing of live cells and the identification of pathogens living in a plaque sample taken from the teeth.) To my amazement, most of my patients had large numbers of microscopic organisms in their mouths, even though their in-office and at-home care was good.

Dr. Trevor Lyons, another pioneer in the microscopic unraveling of periodontal disease, trained as both a periodontist and microbiologist. He broadened the concept that periodontal disease involves oral parasites, such as amoebae, trichomonas and fungus. After reviewing his research, it all made sense. *The true cause of periodontal disease was microorganisms ... germs, and conventional treatment was doing nothing to address the problem!*

In the past dentists were taught that plaque and calculus kept in a germ-free environment have no gum problems, even if they have extensive calculus. They only develop periodontal disease when germs are introduced into their mouths.[1,2]

Periodontal disease is really periodontal infection (PI). PI is caused by microorganisms, and therefore, should be treated like any other infection in the body. The first step in treating PI is to identify the microorganism. Next, an appropriate program of disinfection and cleaning can be instituted, including the use of antimicrobials. Once the infection is under control, surgery may be indicated to repair and reshape damaged tissue. However, removing inflamed tissue without first treating the infection may only provide short-term results.

Why has it taken so long for periodontal disease to be recognized as periodontal infection? Because it takes considerable time for research information to be recognized and integrated into established medical and dental practice.[3,4] For example, in the 1980s a young internist, Barry Marshall, investigated the bacterium known as *Helicobacter pylori*, and proposed it was the cause of peptic ulcers. As valuable as his findings were, it took until the mid-1990s for the medical establishment to finally accept his research as fact.

Equipped with my microscope and my new understanding of the link between periodontal disease and infection, I started making some profound observations. I noted that PI is usually comprised of more than one bug. A more unexpected finding was that the same organisms I found in patients with obvious periodontal infection were also turning up in what appeared to be clean mouths, ones with healthy gums, little plaque and no visible inflammation. Clearly, there was more to preventing PI than brushing and flossing. *I realized that the time to start treating the problem is long before the destruction becomes visible.*

Over the years that followed, it became apparent that proper dental care made a difference in my patients' overall health. For example, with the removal of abscessed teeth associated with unsuccessful root canals, many of my patients reported improvement in their physical condition. Other dental professionals have also acknowledged the connection between the removal of failed root canals and enhanced well-being.[5,6,7]

It was clear to me that what goes on in the mouth is intimately connected to what happens in the rest of the body. As I began learning more about the correlation between PI and major illnesses—such as heart disease, stroke, diabetes, ulcers, obesity, respiratory illness, osteoporosis and complications in pregnancy—I intensified my efforts to establish patient awareness regarding this serious health risk.

How to Use This Book

There is no magic pill to cure PI, but armed with the right techniques and knowledge, you can take the steps necessary to control PI and reap the benefits of significantly improved health. I have written this book for two audiences:

1. Individuals concerned about their own oral and general health; and

2. Medical and dental professionals seeking to improve the care they provide their patients or, as I was, looking for answers to why conventional treatment isn't working.

Depending on your background and objectives, you may choose to read the book sequentially or to jump to the section that interests you most. The next five chapters provide background information on periodontal infection and document its connection to an alarming number of serious health problems. If you are unfamiliar with the pathology of PI or with the latest, state-of-the-art research connecting PI to heart disease and other illnesses, I strongly encourage you to read through those chapters.

The chapters starting with *Diagnosing Periodontal Infection* describe the diagnosis and treatment of PI both in the dental office and at home. If you are familiar with PI research and pathology, or if you have been diagnosed with PI or one of the illnesses with which it is associated, you may wish to begin there. Starting with this chapter will allow you to benefit more quickly from techniques that will help you control the infection.

Throughout the book, I have noted specific studies, journal articles and research papers that support the information I have presented. You can find these listed in the Reference section at the end of the book. Medical and dental professionals may wish to comb through the citations in depth; others may prefer to read the book without using them. There is also a list of definitions in Appendix A, which may help you if you are unfamiliar with a particular term.

When I began my journey almost twenty years ago, I had no idea where it would lead. Now, almost fifteen years after peering through my microscope and coming face-to-face with the enemy, I am surprised at how little has changed in the treatment of periodontal infection, and how many people suffer as a consequence.

So, while I never expected to become an author, I hope you find this book helps you in your own personal quest, whether it is for your health or that of your patients. If so, I have met my objective, and my journey has been worthwhile.

Periodontal Infection: The War in Your Mouth

The word *pocket* is the first word people usually hear from a dentist when there is a problem with their gums. They may also hear *loss of connective tissue attachment,* which means the gums are pulling away from the teeth, creating a pocket. A pocket is just as it sounds—a space that forms between the tooth and the gum. This crevice provides a secure place for bugs to hide. Bugs living at the bottom of a pocket are provided with a protective environment in which they can flourish. (For more detail on pockets and how they are measured, see pages 49 – 50.)

Healthy gums are "stippled," resembling the look of an orange peel in texture. If your gums do not have this look, or are smooth and shiny, you may have a periodontal infection.

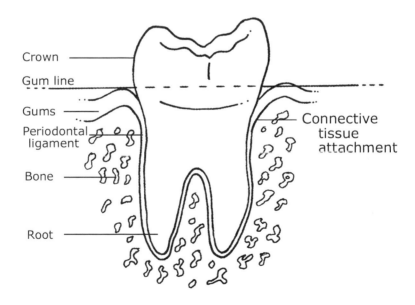

Normal, healthy gums - *The periodontal ligament and bone anchor teeth firmly in place.*

However, healthy-looking gums do not necessarily mean you are bug-free. Certain bugs exist in what appear to be healthy, pocket-free gums; their presence signals the beginning of serious periodontal problems or nutritional deficiencies.

Gum problems:
From the mildest to the most serious

Gingivitis: gums become red and swollen, and bleed easily. The word *gingivitis* comes from *gingiva*, meaning gums, and *itis*, meaning inflammation. *Gingivitis* is an inflammation of the gums. There is generally little or no discomfort at this stage. Gingivitis is usually reversible with professional treatment, coupled with an effective home-care program. Gums may begin to recede, but there is no bone or tooth loss. Pockets are under 3 – 4 mm (3 mm equals 1/8 inch).

Periodontitis is a combination of three Greek words: *peri*, meaning around, *odont*, referring to tooth, and *itis*, which is inflammation. *Periodontitis* is inflammation around the tooth.

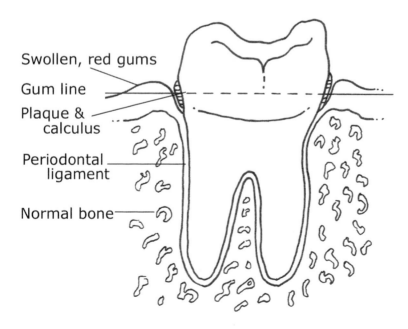

Swollen, red gums

Gum line

Plaque & calculus

Periodontal ligament

Normal bone

Gingivitis - *Gums become red, swollen and bleed easily.*

> *The line between gingivitis and periodontitis is thin. Pockets do not mean that an infection is present, while the absence of pockets does not guarantee that there is no infection.*

Early Periodontitis is the mildest form of periodontal infection. There is a slight loss of connective tissue attachment at this stage. The infection begins to destroy the bone and tissue that support the teeth. There is a sensation that something feels wrong, but it is mild enough to ignore. At this stage brushing and flossing will no longer reach the base of the pockets, which are 3 – 5 mm.

Moderate Periodontitis represents significant bone loss with the teeth beginning to loosen. As bone is lost, more of the tooth is exposed. The ability to arrest the infection becomes more difficult. The root dentin is no longer insulated, and the tooth may become sensitive. Pockets are 5 – 7 mm.

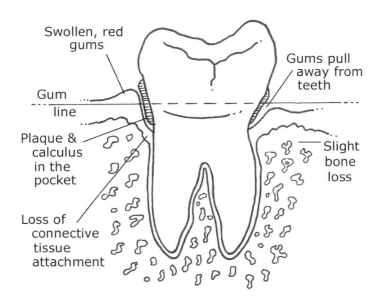

Early Periodontitis - *An early stage periodontal infection begins to destroy the bone and tissue that support the teeth. Gums pull away from the teeth, providing room for bugs to grow.*

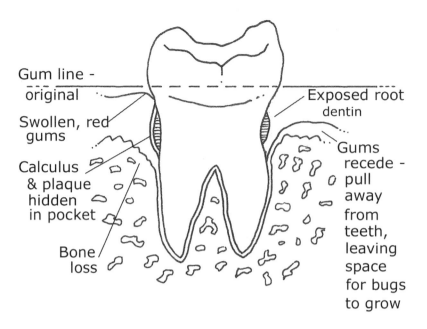

Gum line -
original

Exposed root
dentin

Swollen, red
gums

Calculus
& plaque
hidden
in pocket

Gums
recede -
pull
away
from
teeth,
leaving
space
for bugs
to grow

Bone
loss

Moderate Periodontitis - *Significant bone loss has occurred, and the teeth are beginning to loosen.*

Advanced Periodontitis has devastating bone loss with loosening teeth. If no immediate attention is given, there is a high probability that teeth will become very loose and eventually fall out. Controlling the infection is a major challenge. Sometimes there are periods of significant pain. Pockets are over 6 mm.

Refractory Periodontitis is a rapidly advancing infection that does not respond to typical therapy. This condition includes individuals with recurrent infection at multiple sites and is caused by a combination of factors.

Localized Juvenile Periodontitis normally occurs in adolescents. It is characterized by the rapid loss of bone around one or more permanent teeth. Ironically, youngsters with this infection form very little dental plaque or tartar.

Generalized Juvenile Periodontitis is often considered a disease of young adults, although it can begin around puberty. It is characterized by marked inflammation and heavy accu-

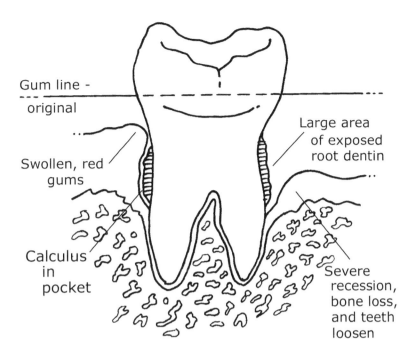

Gum line - original

Large area of exposed root dentin

Swollen, red gums

Calculus in pocket

Severe recession, bone loss, and teeth loosen

Advanced Periodontitis - *Devastating bone loss has occurred, and controlling the infection is a major challenge.*

mulations of plaque and calculus. Pockets can form around the affected teeth, filling with infection. If not treated early, infection can lead to bone loss, which may lead to tooth loss.

The presence of plaque and calculus is another way a dental professional identifies gum problems. Having either plaque or calculus does not mean that you have an infection; however, either of these conditions can encourage microscopic colonization.

Plaque is a sticky, water-repellent coating or bio-film on the teeth and gums. It is composed of food debris and over 300 forms of bacteria, viruses and fungi and their waste products. Plaque left on your teeth over 24 hours forms a matrix that attracts dissolved minerals in the saliva. *This precipitation of mineral salts is the beginning of calculus; this is why it is very important to thoroughly brush and floss your teeth at least once a day.*

Calculus (tartar) is the hardened, porous buildup of mineral salts and dead bacteria. It mainly accumulates on the inside of the lower front teeth and the outside of the upper molars, near the saliva ducts. It may be many different colors: yellow, brown, black, orange or green, depending on how it developed. The main problem is that calculus forms in places that routine brushing and flossing do not reach, making calculus a haven for bacteria.

Saliva is the mineral-rich fluid that keeps the teeth hard, lubricates the mouth, and provides digestive enzymes. But saliva also plays an important role in a healthy mouth. It impairs the growth of bacteria by washing them away, along with acidic bacterial waste products that can dissolve tooth structure. Dry mouth can cause more than just an uncomfortable feeling. Dryness means that you do not have enough saliva, the mouth's natural protective fluid. Unfortunately, there are many prescription drugs today that list dry mouth as a possible side effect.

Health Challenges & Periodontal Infection

The Big Health Picture

The National Institute of Dental Research states that 75% of the adult population has moderate to advanced periodontal infection, 90% has some

> *If your dentist says that you have no periodontal problems, your dentist probably isn't looking hard enough.*

form of gingivitis, and 30% of children have moderate PI. According to the National Institute of Health, "the incidence of PI exceeds 70% in the 30 – 44 age groups and 90% in the 55 – 64 age group… the prevalence and severity of PI will increase as the life expectancy of the population and retention of teeth increase."[8,9]

Why treat the first few inches of the digestive tract, which begins at your mouth, differently from the rest of your body? A physician would consider the presence of a few bugs (e.g. protozoa, amoebae or spirochetes) anywhere in the body as a serious health threat. However, some dental professionals consider having these organisms in the mouth only a minor localized problem.

Present research overwhelmingly supports the assertion that PI affects the rest of the body in dramatic ways.[10,11,12] Germs enter the bloodstream from infected gum tissue, sometimes just by chewing. Routine oral-health practices such as flossing, using a toothpick, or even brushing can open pathways for bugs. I am not recommending abandoning these good oral-hygiene practices; rather, I am illustrating how easy it is for bacteria to enter the blood stream.

If you have an unhealthy mouth,
you have an unhealthy body!

The Surgeon General's Report on Oral Health: Implications on Research and Education stresses the seriousness of the connection between PI and many systemic diseases. Furthermore, the report emphasizes that problems generated from the mouth must be considered by all members of the medical profession.[13] Other research associates PI with over forty diseases, including heart disease, stroke and diabetes. The sheer number of studies that directly or indirectly examine the oral-systemic link is substantial.[14,15]

Jack Caton, D.D.S., President of the American Academy of Periodontology states, "Avoiding periodontal disease is not just important for keeping teeth for a lifetime, but also in keeping the rest of the body healthy." Dr. James Beck, co-director of The Center for Oral and Systemic Diseases at the University of North Carolina Dental School, adds "There are associations... we are beginning to understand the biology better than we did before."[16]

A study from the Michigan School of Dentistry goes even further, associating poor dental health with "early death from any cause."[17] *Parade Magazine*, March 26, 2000 has an article entitled "Keep Your Gums Healthy—And Your Heart Will Benefit." The word is definitely getting out.

A Dental Products Report Survey from April 1999 stated that 86% of the dentists questioned believed that their patients have an increased awareness of PI, but of this 86%, only 4% were using effective techniques to evaluate this major health concern.

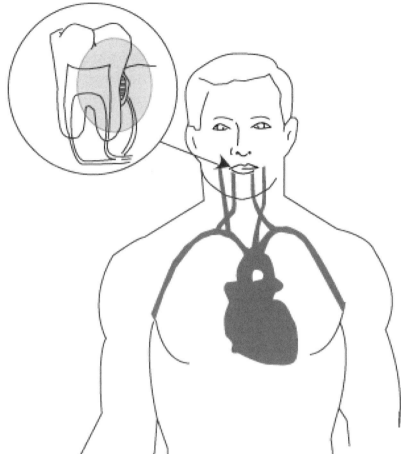

From your gums to your heart - *One theory explaining the connection between PI and heart disease is that oral bacteria enter the bloodstream, attaching to fatty plaques in coronary arteries and contributing to clot formation.*

Heart Disease

There is increasing awareness in medical literature that coronary heart disease is linked not only to hereditary and nutritional factors, but that it also has an infectious origin.[18,19, 20, 21]

Heart attacks and strokes are often associated with fatty deposits called arthromeres. Outstanding research done at the Department of Oral Biology, School of Dental Medicine, State University of NY at Buffalo (SUNYAB) discovered that fatty deposits contain DNA remnants from a variety of periodontal microorganisms. The study concluded that periodontal microorganisms were present in the plaque inside arteries, where they might play a role in the development and progression of certain kinds of heart disease.[22]

A second study of 10,000 adults, ages seventeen and over, found that persons with PI have increased levels of the blood-clotting factor fibrinogen. (An elevated fibrinogen level is known to be an independent risk factor for cardiovascular disease.) The research team at SUNYAB said bacteria from PI appeared to have entered the blood, possibly spurring the body to produce such factors as fibrinogen, which can cause blocked arteries.[23]

Adding to this problem were two gene patterns, H2H2 and H2H1, which produce higher levels of fibrinogen. Since the production of fibrinogen can be stimulated by infection, people with these gene patterns produced higher levels of this clotting factor, thus putting them at an even higher risk for heart disease.[24]

Furthermore, Dr. Robert Genco from SUNYAB identified several types of periodontal bacteria as causing damage to the heart: *B. forsythias*, *P. gingivalis*, and *C. recta*. He found that the risk of heart problems was 200 – 300% higher in persons with one or more of these oral bacteria.[25]

At the University of Michigan (UM), Dr. Walter Loesche reported that patients with periodontitis were much more likely to have cardiovascular disease, even after accounting for all other causes, such as smoking, cholesterol, triglycerides and obesity. Total mortality was two and one-half times greater in patients with PI.[26] In a six-year study, a sample of 44,119 male health professionals (58% of whom were dentists) with no major pre-existing conditions reported significant correlation between PI and coronary heart disease.[27]

Another study reported that patients between the ages of 30 – 40 who showed evidence of bone loss around teeth were

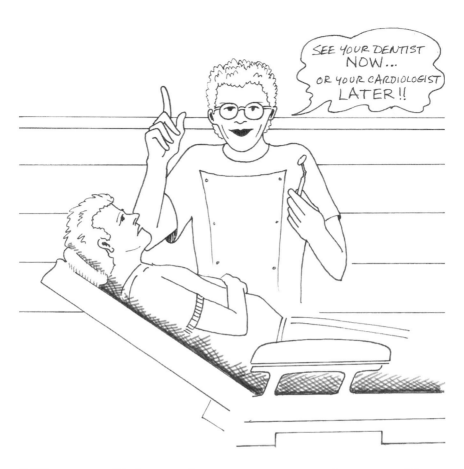

50% more likely to have a coronary heart problem. Furthermore, fatal heart disease was twice as common in those with PI.[28]

Researchers at the University of North Carolina, Chapel Hill, (UNC) conducted a long-term study involving 1,147 men. The study concluded that having PI increases the risk for coronary heart disease by 150%, for fatal coronary heart disease by 190%, and for stroke by 280%. It was found that heart attack survivors with PI also have a greater risk of suffering a second heart attack.[29]

UNC also added that heart-attack survivors who have advanced PI are more likely to have elevated blood levels of C-reactive-factor protein (CRP), an inflammatory protein associated with heart disease. Further research noted that CRP levels were directly related to the severity of the PI.[30]

Other research from UNC verifying the "Heart-PI connection" comes from the Third National Health and Nutritional Examination Survey (NHANES III) of 5,564 people forty years and older. The results clearly support findings from previous studies of a strong association between PI and coronary heart disease.[31]

Scientists at the University of Minnesota have studied the bacterium *streptococcus sanguis* ("strep"), a common tooth-plaque bacteria, in an effort to further understand the correlation between PI and heart attacks. Initial tests found that this particular strain of strep caused human blood platelet cells to form clots. To test the theory, they introduced small amounts of strep into the bloodstream of rabbits. Within three minutes of introducing the bacterium, the animals' heart rates, breathing and blood pressures all increased dramatically.[32]

Electrocardiograms (EKGs) of the rabbits also revealed abnormal heartbeat patterns. Further analysis showed that these aberrant beats were a direct result of inadequate amounts of oxygen being received by the heart muscle. This scenario is precisely what occurs just before humans experience a heart attack.[33]

Obviously, not all individuals have a heart attack every time their gums bleed. Under ideal circumstances, the bacteria that enter the bloodstream are removed quickly by the immune system. But for people who already have serious heart disease or a compromised immune system, the risk is much greater.

The Department of Oral Biology, University of Florida at Gainesville, tested in vitro the ability of three periodontal pathogens to invade the cells that coat the inside of the artery (endothelial cells) and the smooth muscle cells of the coronary artery. The study demonstrated that specific species and strains of bacteria do invade coronary artery cells at significant levels. This was the first documented study of its kind to establish how oral microorganisms invade human primary cell cultures of the circulatory system.[34]

At the Helsinki University Central Hospital, Finland, doctors followed the medical history of 9,760 patients for fourteen years. They confirmed that those with the most severe dental infections at the beginning of the study had a 25% increased risk of developing coronary heart disease, *especially men under 50 years of age.*[35]

Another Finnish study compared the degree of coronary artery damage to the severity of gum disease in 100 patients.[36] In both studies the association remained valid after adjustment for age, social class, smoking, cholesterol, socio-economic levels and the presence of diabetes.[37]

Heart disease is not the only serious systemic illness that research has correlated with gum disease. A diverse list of adverse health conditions have also been linked to the presence of PI, including stroke, diabetes, ulcers, obesity, respiratory illnesses, osteoporosis and complications in pregnancy.

Stroke

The First National Health and Nutrition Examination Survey and its follow-up represents the first major study correlating cerebrovascular accidents (strokes) with PI. The study comprised 9,962 adults, ages 25 to 74, categorized from no PI to significant PI. The results were astounding: having PI represented more than a 200% greater risk for total strokes and, in particular, non-bleeding strokes. The risk was the same for African-Americans and Caucasians.[38]

Arnin Grau, M.D., of the Department of Neurology at the University of Heidelberg, Germany discovered that poor dental status resulting from chronic dental and bone infection was

> *"In stroke cases, only the dental factor is causative and significant."*
>
> Arnin Grau, M.D.
> Department of Neurology
> University of Heidelberg

associated with a stroke increase of two and one-half times over non-PI patients. In fact, stroke patients are three times more likely to have PI. "In stroke cases, only the dental factor is causative and significant."[39]

Diabetes (Diabetes Mellitus)

Previously, it was assumed that the association between PI and diabetes was the diabetic patient's compromised ability to respond to infectious challenges. Therefore, they were predisposed to bacterial infections such as PI.

However, now the opposite possibility should be considered. Dr. Robert Genco, chairman of Oral Biology Department at SUNYAB, said, "Diabetics are at a higher risk for periodontal disease." His studies show that treating PI may reduce a diabetic's blood sugar levels.[40,41]

One study of insulin users compared diabetic adults with mild PI to those with severe PI. Periodontal examinations

> *Diabetes mellitus is a collection of health problems that are characterized by a decline in or lack of insulin production. Unfortunately about 50% of this type of diabetes goes unrecognized.*[48]

were performed at the beginning of the study with follow-up over eleven years. The diabetic condition remained constant. The summary over the follow-up period showed the incidence of stroke, angina and heart failure was four times higher with the severe PI group, as compared to the mild PI group.

Another study tested the hypothesis that severe PI increases the concentration of blood sugar in serum in persons with type 2 diabetes.[42] The results of this study and others show that PI is associated with a significant worsening of the diabetic condition.[43,44,45] Undiagnosed diabetes should be considered when a patient has advanced periodontitis in the absence of other risk factors.[46,47,48]

Stomach Ulcers and H. Pylori

Helicobacter pylori (*H. pylori*) is a species of bacteria that is found in the stomach lining of 50% of all Americans and has been associated with stomach ulcers and stomach cancer. Dr. Barry Marshall proved, by voluntarily self-administering the bacteria into his body and then treating himself with antibiotics, that these "spiral-shaped bugs" caused ulcers. Furthermore, it was discovered that *H. pylori* was also present in infected gum tissue.[49]

Even when *H. pylori* was eliminated from the stomach with antibiotic therapy, it was not completely eradicated from the mouth, where it continues to grow in colonies deep within periodontal pockets. These pockets could be a source of re-infection for the stomach.[50]

Obesity and Weight Loss

Researchers from the School of Dental Medicine at SUNYAB have found that the inability to lose weight is significantly related to PI through the path of insulin resistance. (Insulin resistance is when cells do not absorb insulin from the blood stream efficiently.) Dr. Sara Grossi, clinical assistant professor of oral biology, director of the UB Periodontal Disease Research Center states, "Acute infections cause metabolic disturbances, and periodontal disease is one of humankind's most common chronic infections. In this case, we think bacteria from gum disease may interfere with fat metabolism, leading to elevated LDL cholesterol and total cholesterol."[51]

Statistics correlate obesity and PI. Results obtained from the Third National Health and Nutrition Examination (NHANES III) show that overweight people with the highest levels of insulin resistance are 50% more likely to have severe PI compared to overweight people with low insulin resistance.[52]

Dr. O. A'cbay and his team discovered that *H. pylori* in the stomach triggers the release of the hormone gastrin. Gastrin acts to stimulate the pancreas to release insulin, causing hyperinsulinemia, a serious condition that may not only result in diabetic complications and obesity but also put the heart at risk. Further studies are warranted to investigate whether eliminating *H. pylori* in the stomach can help in weight reduction.[53]

Pneumonia and Respiratory Diseases

Bacterial respiratory infections may be acquired by inhaling fine droplets of oral fluids from the mouth and throat. These droplets contain germs, which can breed and multiply within the lungs. It is recognized that pneumonia and lung abscesses can result from the same bacteria that cause PI. Dental plaque would seem to be a logical source of these bacteria, especially in patients with PI.[54]

The occurrence of advanced PI in patients with pneumonia has been estimated to be well over 50%. Parasites, viruses, fungi and bacteria cause this life threatening disease; especially susceptible are elderly and immune-compromised individuals. Pneumonia is the number one cause of death in nursing homes and the leading cause of death in those over 65.[55]

Studies from the University of California point to the link between poor oral health and respiratory disease, especially chronic respiratory disease in non-smokers. The same research shows significant correlation between PI and risk of chronic obstructive pulmonary disease.[56]

Pregnancy

Pre-term, low, birth weight babies (PTLBW)

Researchers at the University of North Carolina (UNC) have made an enormous contribution to understanding the correlation between PI and pre-term, low-birth-weight babies (PTLBW). Many factors, including hormones and locally acting inflammatory chemical messengers, play a key role in regulating the onset of labor, cervical opening, contractions and delivery. An infectious process appears to trigger either early labor or a premature rupture of membranes by placing undue stress on the immune system.[57]

> *PI may be as serious a risk to a pregnant woman's fetus as are the use of alcohol, drugs and tobacco.*

The study significantly correlated the presence of four organisms associated with mature dental plaque and progressing PI to the probability of having a PTLBW. The conclusion was that, after accounting for all of the normally accepted obstetric risk factors, mothers with PI have a significantly higher number of PTLBW.[58,59,60]

Other studies support these findings. Mothers with PTLBW, who were otherwise considered low risk, were suspected to have PI as the cause of early delivery.[61] Another study determined that a woman was seven times more likely to have a PTLBW if severe PI was present. PI may be as serious a risk to a pregnant woman's fetus as are the use of alcohol, drugs and tobacco.[62]

Marjorie Jeffcoat, D.M.D., Department of Periodontics at the University of Alabama at Birmingham School of Dentistry stated, "...the trend for pre-term birth was observed in women with as little as two sites (of PI)."[63]

F. nucleatum is a common bacteria found in oral plaque. The Department of Obstetrics and Gynecology at Duke

University isolated *F. nucleatum* (the most frequently isolated species from amniotic fluid) and correlated its presence with PTLBW, demonstrating that PI from the mouth to amniotic fluid not only was possible but could very well lead to delivery problems.[64]

Further studies in "The Journal of Infectious Immunity" were conducted on hamsters. When maternal hamsters were exposed to a common oral pathogen, such as *P. gingivalis*, they experienced stressed delivery.[65,66]

Osteoporosis

Dental researchers have established a connection between PI and bone disease. A study at SUNYAB reviewed the medical records of 2,599 postmenopausal women and found that women who had osteoporosis of the hip were two times more likely to have loose teeth and PI than women with healthy hip bones.[67]

A study conducted at the University of Toronto Department of Periodontics suggests that periodontal pathogens, such as *P. gingivalis*, might contribute to bone loss in PI not only by stimulating reabsorption but, possibly, by inhibiting bone formation directly.[68]

Researchers are starting to use bone scans to compare the bone density of the hip to that of the bone surrounding the teeth. Preliminary results indicate that, as dental bone density decreases, so does hip bone density. Further studies are warranted.[69]

Bugs Versus Us

The immune system is a network of cells and organs that work together to defend the body against attacks by bugs, aka: microorganisms, bacteria, viruses, parasites and fungi. Because the dark, damp human mouth provides an ideal environment for these microorganisms to flourish, it is the immune system's job to carry out search and destroy missions.[70]

There are more than 300 species of bacteria alone that have been isolated from periodontal pockets, but only a few that actually cause periodontal destruction. These few "bad bugs" prove the principle of survival of the fittest.[71]

The fact that we cannot see, touch or hear microorganisms does not mean that they do not exist and are not challenging our immune system for their right to survive.[72] The battlefield of microorganisms can be clearly viewed through a phase-contrast microscope. The activity, speed and intensity of these microscopic armies demonstrate vitality that all of us would be envious to possess.

A video monitor attached to the microscope brings the viewer into the battle and immediately displays throngs of microscopic invaders waiting at the gate. These attackers appear to have a collective conscious. They show purpose in their activity—sometimes working as a team, sometimes working alone, always at a frenetic pace.

Organisms that are considered to be bad possess the ability to:

1. Colonize (create a home and multiply);
2. Evade and disrupt protective defense mechanisms;
3. Produce substances that directly initiate tissue destruction and cause the progression of infection.[73,74]

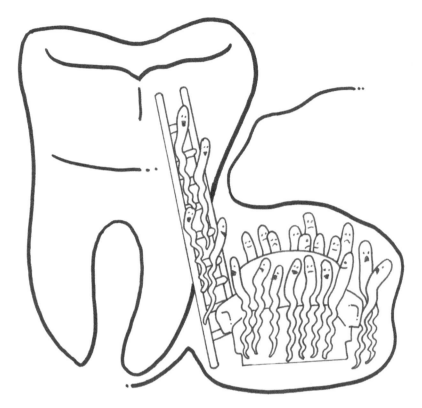

Home Sweet Pocket - *In advanced PI, spirochetes can line up and pulse in a wavelike motion*

Periodontal pockets and tissue have their own ecosystem. For example, a common pathogen, *P. gingivalis*, can encapsulate itself to resist defensive antibodies. As soon as these bugs have a protective shield, they start invading deeper into the pocket. Once settled in, they are very good at fortifying their position to have better on-going access to us, the host.[75,76,77,78]

This encapsulation ability creates a strong defensive posture, which makes these organisms difficult to eradicate once they have gained a foothold. Perhaps this is why conventional root scraping therapy used alone has limited success; it temporarily destroys the bugs' homes but does not get rid of them.

Procedures like root planing provide a short period of relief but allow the bugs to rebuild and repopulate as strong and virulent as ever.[79] Aggressive root planing removes the outer covering of the root called cementum. Cementum is a natural barrier that prevents pathogens from invading the root and reaching the pulp of the tooth. Once the cementum is gone, the tooth is more vulnerable to invasion.[80]

The Immune System Breakdown

The good, the bad and the ugly

Under normal circumstances the immune system recognizes and destroys enemy invaders. This is **good**. For example, when you cut your hand, it heals easily after a little red inflammation.[81,82]

But pathogens are capable of many evasive maneuvers. For example, by producing their own toxins and enzymes, certain microorganisms are capable of destroying most of the body's defense systems. Consequently, defensive cells may either never be activated, or they may activate systems that cause significant inflammation.[83,84,85,86,87]

> *When inflammation is raging, it increases swelling and redness, allowing for an even greater penetration of bacteria and toxins.*

Once our initial defensive system is pierced, other destructive systems are initiated. When the body realizes invaders are still present, it kicks production of defensive cells into high gear. Unfortunately, this causes an even more serious inflammation to develop. Now the defensive cells are **bad** because they become as destructive as they were initially protective.

Defensive cells, even after dying, release large quantities of potent chemical messengers called cytokines into the local area. Some cytokines are capable of degrading gum tissue.

Other chemical messengers promote the release of enzymes called MMPs (matrix metalloproteinases). These enzymes destroy bone, and bone reabsorption begins.[88,89,90]

The most important inflammatory enzyme is collagenase. It is responsible for the breakdown of collagen, the foundation of all our connective tissue.

---

*And now **the ugly**… this reabsorption process causes teeth to get loose and fall out.[91]*

From a personal perspective this is a devastating event; however, from a self-preservation viewpoint, this is the way the body rids itself of a life threatening infection. If all else fails, **as it does with a splinter, the body just eliminates it! Once the tooth comes out, the gums heal, and the infection disappears.**

What about a moderate case of gingivitis?

How about the bad bugs' less virulent cousins, which can cause a mild gingival irritation? Most dentists think that this is a condition to monitor but not to be overly concerned about.

The continuous production of these not-so-toxic bacteria may result in swelling (edema) and tissue vulnerability, however. This provides an excellent home and environment for the more destructive pathogens, analogous to a crumbling wall around a castle. As long as the enemy stays away, there is peace. But once an aggressive foe enters, there is little resistance.[92]

How Our Immune System Works

The immune system is designed to protect our bodies from invading microorganisms, as well as toxic by-products of our own metabolism. The immune system, rather than drugs or doctors, is the main avenue of protection and cure we have. It is worthwhile to understand the basic principles of this complex system. From colds to cancer, no illness can be combated without it.

The following description of the structure and function of the basic components of the immune system is non-technical and is designed to translate scientific jargon into language that is understandable.

General Immune System

Our body's defense depends on several systems working together to protect us against our enemies. The general system works like a sanitation department. The workers in this clean-up crew are called *macrophages*. (See illustration on following page.) They do their cleaning by eating and digesting the enemy. Macrophages number in the millions and are located throughout the body.

Macrophages seek-out, surround, take in, breakdown, and spit out or transport invaders, toxins and the body's own wastes. This process is known as *phagocytosis*. The general immune system is accompanied and aided by the specific immune system.[93,94,95]

Specific Immune System

The specific immune system starts with primitive stem cells produced in the bone marrow. These cells differentiate into T-cells and B-cells. The T-cells get their special instructions in the thymus, hence the 'T'. The T-cells further differentiate into helper, suppressor and natural killer cells. The B-cells were named for an area of a bird's intestine called the *bursa*, where B-cells were first isolated. The area of the body where B-cells get their instructions is not known with certainty, but it is most likely in the

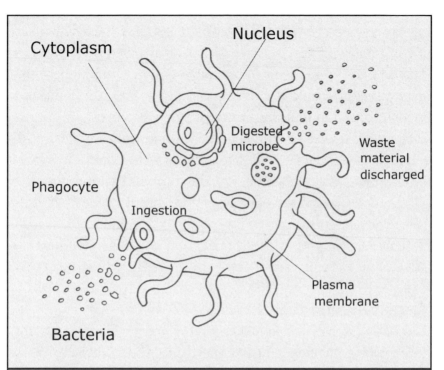

Macrophages *are the clean-up crew for the body's immune system. They seek out and consume or transport invaders, toxins and the body's own waste.*

spleen or intestines. B-cells control the defense against specific microorganisms. There are many other named cells, but only the mechanism of the B-cells will be discussed.

To work effectively, B-cells need the cooperation of many other cells. B-cells communicate by direct physical contact and also by releasing chemical messengers to summon their allies.

In order to have room to store all of the cells needed for an effective defense against millions of possible invaders, the immune system only keeps a few of each specific defensive cell ready at any given time. Enemies are identified by an appendage on their cell walls called an *antigen*. This antigen can be recognized by the defensive system in two ways.

First, B-cells continuously release a small amount of Y-shaped substances called *antibodies* into the body's fluids. An antibody has one long leg and two shorter claw arms and untiringly feels the shapes of all the substances it contacts. If the claw arms fit the antigen, the arms slip into place around the antigen and remain attached. This forms what is called an *immune complex*.

Immune complexes transmit signals indicating that macrophages should come and destroy them. Antibodies are only supposed to fit antigens on foreign substances. This is generally quite a good system; however, at times small errors result, and serious consequences develop. It is possible for the formation of immune complexes to get out of control. Depending on what tissue or source of antigen is involved, an autoimmune disease can develop.

Second, if a B-cell encounters its specific antigen on an enemy, it can link up to the invader directly. This triggers a reaction in the B-cell to make *plasma cells*. Each plasma cell is a factory for producing its specific antibody. Descended from a single B-cell, plasma cells manufacture millions of identical antibodies and pour them into the blood stream to mark invaders. After the invaders are overcome, the suppressor T-cells eliminate unused antibodies and the macrophages get to work.

Assisting these defensive cells is a cascade of naturally occurring proteins and glycoproteins called the *complement system*. One of its main functions is the bursting (*lysis*) of unwanted cells, such as early cancer cells, bacteria or envelope-coated viruses.

The complement cascade is similar to a row of upright dominoes that knock each other over when the first one falls. The first complement protein attaches onto an antibody/antigen combination on the enemy cell. Each protein tags the next protein in line until all proteins are turned on. The last protein in the cascade punctures a hole and inserts a cylinder in the enemy cell wall.[96]

Another function is the marking of unwanted cellular debris for removal by the macrophages by coating the particles with complement proteins that fit the receptors in the macrophage cells. The result is protection of the host by regulating the inflammatory and immune responses. Unfortunately, when this process gets out of control the consequences include inflammation, redness, warmth, swelling and pain.[97]

Who Gets the Bugs?

T he microorganisms that cause PI are always looking for a hospitable environment in which to set up house-keeping. But why do some people escape their attack while others do not?

> *"In my lifetime, advances in life expectancy are primarily due to an increase in hygiene."*
>
> *Detrick Klinghart M.D.*

There are a number of factors that determine an individual's propensity to develop periodontal infection, including nutrition, genetics, improper tooth alignment, and the use of tobacco, alcohol and certain medications. We will cover those factors below.

Perhaps the most important factor, though, is oral hygiene. Individuals who have dirty mouths are more likely to get PI. A sound program of home care is the first step in protecting yourself.

Individuals who are disabled or, for other reasons, unable to provide a good home care program should seek frequent professional help from a dental hygienist. It's a small price to pay to protect your health.

Nutrition

Researchers at SUNYAB found that people who consume less than the recommended dietary allowance (RDA) of Vitamin C have higher rates of PI. They analyzed Vitamin C intakes and PI indicators in 12,419 U.S. adults and found that patients who consumed less than the recommended 60 mg. per day were at nearly 1½ times the risk of developing severe gingivitis as those who consumed three times the RDA. "The relationship between Vitamin C and PI is likely due to Vitamin C's role in maintaining and repairing healthy connective tissue, along with its antioxidant properties… PI is an inflammatory disorder that increases tissue damage and loss. Since Vitamin C is known as a powerful scavenger of reactive oxygen species (free radicals), low levels of dietary Vitamin C may compromise the body's ability to neutralize these tissue destructive oxidants."[98]

Good nutrition is critical in the fight against PI. A weak immune system can make it harder for the body to fight infection. Certain nutrients are essential for a healthy immune system to thrive. The Third National Health and Nutrition Examination (NHANES III) study from 9,862 individuals reveals how important good nutrition and supplementation is to dental health. The most impressive statistic was that low selenium levels increased the risk of PI by thirteen times. Low levels of vitamins A and C also increased the risk of gum disease.[99]

Antioxidants are vital for combating PI. Free radicals are released as a result of killing bacteria. Increased levels of antioxidants are required to overcome free radical damage.

Free radicals: Friend or Foe?

Free radicals are potent toxic substances released by white blood cells when fighting infection. They are the body's main weapon. Free radicals are capable of eating holes in bacterial membranes.

A free radical occurs when an oxygen atom loses one of its electrons. If the oxygen atom tries to replace the missing electron with an electron from a molecule in a cell wall, a new free radical is created. This process can begin a chain reaction leading to disintegration of the target cell.

If not controlled, over-release of free radicals can be damaging to surrounding tissue. Antioxidants give up electrons to neutralize free radicals without becoming harmful themselves. Infection depletes the body's supply of antioxidants. Supplementation with antioxidants restores balance.

When antioxidant levels drop significantly, the ability to control inflammation is compromised.

Genetics

Genetics plays a role in PI. Certain individuals with specific genetic patterns (genotype) make more Interleukin 1 (IL-1), an inflammatory mediator (cytokine), in response to bacterial plaque. This high level of IL-1 results in rapid and extensive damage to the surrounding tissues.[100]

A study by Komman and colleagues found that 67% of patients with severe PI had the IL-1 genotype. Patients can be tested for the presence of IL-1 genotype by laboratory analysis of a finger-stick drop of blood.[101]

Another group that are at increased risk for developing PI have defective white cells. These individuals cannot even begin to launch an effective fight.[102]

Medications

The use of medications may limit a person's ability to fight PI. While beneficial for a specific health challenge, certain medications may reduce the power of white blood cells to function effectively.[103,104,105] A different problem has been observed with people using calcium channel-blockers. In one study 43.6% of patients receiving the calcium channel-blocking agent nifedipine were reported to experience gingival overgrowth. This creates pseudo pockets, where bugs can find a sheltered home.[106]

Tobacco Use

Drs. Scott Tomar and Samira Asma examined oral health results from the NHANES III survey involving more than 12,000 individuals, minimum age eighteen, from 1988 – 1994. Their findings are critical. They outline in their report that 50% of the cases of PI affecting U.S. adults may be attributable to cigarette smoking. In current smokers, the occurrence may be as high as 75%.[107]

Smoking is detrimental to gum tissue. It weakens the natural ability of white cells to fight infection by preventing oxygen and nutrients from reaching the gingival tissue. The Department of Oral Microbiology at Malmo, Sweden, found that smoking alters the environment in the periodontal pocket, making it more susceptible to bacteria.[108]

In addition, tars and other chemicals found in smoke, which are thin and difficult to see, precipitate on teeth and root surfaces just like they do on the inside of a windshield of a smoker's car. This same type of film deposited in the mouth leaves the area vulnerable to attack.[109]

An interesting note is that bone and tooth loss, PI, and oral sores in the mouth may more strongly motivate patients to stop using tobacco than does the threat of lung cancer or cardiovascular disease. Also, eleven years after quitting, former smokers' likelihood of having PI is about the same as those who never smoked. It pays to quit.[110,111]

If you think that smoking isn't your problem, consider this: results from the NHANES III study people compiled from 1988 – 1994 found that persons exposed to second-hand, or passive, smoking had a significantly increased risk of serious PI than those not exposed. This health threat remained substantial after adjusting for age, gender, race, education, income and diabetes.[112]

Alcohol Use

The NHANES III study analyzed random data from 6,492 subjects between the ages of twenty and ninety to determine the link between alcohol consumption and PI. As alcohol consumption increases from five to twenty drinks per week, so the risk of PI increases in direct proportion from 10% to 40%.[113]

Alcohol also depletes B vitamins and protein components necessary for healing. The reason for such high correlation may be the body's inability to fight infection and form new bone.[114]

Alignment of Teeth

Improper tooth positioning, such as crowded and/or rotated teeth, can result in the creation of food traps, producing breeding grounds for bugs. Teeth that hit incorrectly can cause excessive or improper pressure on other teeth resulting in pain or loose teeth. The area around these injured teeth are more susceptible to PI. Imagine a stake in the earth that is constantly being twisted and leaned on. After awhile, the ground moves away from the stake making it loose. The same thing happens with a tooth, except now the "loose ground," gum tissue, is vulnerable to a bacterial invasion.

Pregnancy Gingivitis

Changing hormonal levels create this condition, and it usually disappears after the birth. However, the current research on the link between PI and PTLBW babies is so significant that all pregnant women should have regular dental check-ups throughout their pregnancies.

Braces

Braces are a form of man-made calculus. The brackets and wires effectively block toothbrush bristles from scrubbing away plaque. Fortunately, most orthodontics is done on teenagers who have good immune systems that keep the bug population under control. However, an electric toothbrush and irrigator should be standard equipment to insure that no permanent damage takes place during this vulnerable time. This is especially true for adults undergoing this type of procedure.

People With Good Teeth

There are growing numbers of people who have escaped the ravages of dental decay. In youth these people are blessed. They have perfect teeth, with little effort directed towards brushing and flossing. However, these people are often infected with pathogens that cause PI, because they rarely go to the dentist and often have lax home care standards. Further complicating this situation is the fact that, even when notified of PI, these people tend to stay in a state of disbelief that anything can be dentally wrong with them.

Infections Are Contagious!

PI is easily transmitted. The majority of periodontal microorganisms are shared between family members. This logically points out the importance of treating the entire family. The Journal of Dental Research, using Dr. W.J. Loesche's BANA test, found that children whose parents were infected by the bacteria recognized in the test were almost ten times more likely to have the same bacteria in their mouths. Children whose parents had clinical evidence of PI were twelve times (1200%) more likely to have the same bacteria[115,116,117,118,119]

If you have diagnosed PI, there is a very good chance that other members of your family, including your children, are also infected.[120,121] To prevent this, members of a family in which someone has PI should use separate eating utensils, including glasses and straws. Make a concerted effort not to exchange saliva by any means, such as wetting a pacifier for a baby. People can also get infected or reinfected at the workplace, so similar precautions apply.

Animals get PI, too! One of my patients had very stubborn PI that my hygienist could not get under control. Finally, a sample of plaque was taken from the family dog, and the culprit was found![122]

Super-Germs and Antibiotic Use

When and why you don't respond to antibiotics!

We are approaching a crisis that will affect the health of millions of people: the emergence of antibiotic-resistant bacteria.[123] During the 1970s, infectious diseases appeared to be under control. Yet, in the last twenty years the re-emergence of infection-related illnesses, due to what have been labeled *super-germs* has been alarming.[124]

How Is This Happening?

Along with other factors, such as the overuse of antibiotics, mercury/silver amalgam fillings are seriously implicated in the creation of super-germs. Researchers at the University of Georgia and the Faculty of Medicine at the University of Calgary made a startling discovery. Extensive testing was done on the intestinal bacteria of subjects who had silver-amalgam fillings (50% mercury) in their mouths. Data showed that mercury from these fillings was also found in the intestinal tract. The mercury residing in the intestines would normally be poisonous to intestinal bacteria. However, since bacteria are able to adapt easily, the bacterial population, in an information swap or gene exchange, produced a new generation that can withstand the toxic environment created by the mercury.

Their further analysis revealed a disturbing fact: that the subject's new generation of intestinal bacteria were now capable of easily developing resistance to antibiotics.[125,126,127]

So there is a possibility that, if you have amalgam fillings, antibiotics may not be effective for you.

Overuse of Antibiotics

Antibiotics have been a blessing to modern society since the introduction of penicillin. The current thought regarding many infections is to drown them in antibiotics. Unfortunately, this way of thinking is making life-saving antibiotics useless against certain bugs.

Antibiotics often destroy only weak bacteria, leaving the strong alive. With weaker family members killed, the remaining bugs become resistant to the antibiotic that wiped out their puny cousins and have more room to expand into new strains of super-bugs. Basically, bacteria are getting it together much faster than drug companies can produce new antibiotics to destroy them.[128,129,130,131]

Bacteria are capable of rapid genetic improvement to out-wit any change in their environment, including the newest

---

"When antibiotics were introduced, some hoped that they might put an end to bacterial disease. The track record, as of the mid-1940s, bolstered this lofty expectation, at least for those who did not bother to consider evolution. Those who did, however, sounded an alarm almost from the beginning of the antibiotic era. The discoverer of penicillin, Alexander Fleming, warned in the late 1940s that antibiotics might soon lose their effectiveness through the evolution of antibiotic resistance. Another Nobel lau-reate, Joshua Lederberg, voiced a similar warning during the early 1950s. But the alarm went largely unheeded.[147]

---

antibiotics. They are able to pass along these good genes in extra genetic bundles called *plasmids*. Bacteria can also fuse with other species of bacteria and share their resistant traits.[132]

Antibiotics (which means "against life") destroy friendly bacteria as well as the targeted bacteria. *Probiotics* (which means "for life") are friendly bacteria that are essential to the health of our immune systems. When probiotics are growing and flourishing in the intestines, harmful bacteria pass right through the system without doing any damage. After antibiotics destroy bad and good bacteria alike, aggressive, harmful bacteria can repopulate the intestines more easily.

The widespread and indiscriminant use of antibiotics is a serious health concern. We have listed below some of the more common examples of such use.

Antibiotics Prescribed for Colds and Flu

Antibiotics are still being given routinely at the first sign of a cold or flu, even though research has shown that most of these illnesses are viral. *Antibiotics are useless against viruses.* Jon Rosenberg, M.D., states, "Resistance problems emerge when increasing numbers of patients' infections fail to respond to treatment."[133]

The highly virulent staphylococcus became resistant in 1975 to everything but Vancomycin, and some feel that it will soon overcome this last antibiotic stronghold.[134]

Antibacterial Soaps

The new entrant in anti-germ warfare is anti-bacterial hand-and-body soaps. Until recently, people used soap and water to wash away bacteria. Now the goal is to kill bacteria with anti-bacterial compounds. The Soap and Detergent Association reports that approximately 45% of the hand and body wash products contain anti-bacterial compounds. Unfortunately, the same selective breeding of the fittest occurs in these anti-bacterial products that kills the weakest and leaves the strongest.[135]

Antibiotics in Animal Feed

The U.S. remains one of the last major countries that still allow the addition of antibiotics to animal feed, simply for the purpose of maximizing weight gain. In 1985, animals were fed 18 million pounds of antibiotics. In 1992, there were approximately 50,000 pounds of antibiotics sprayed just on U.S. fruit trees. This widespread misuse is contributing to the breeding of new strains of germs.[136]

The Pre-medication Controversy

What bleeds out, bleeds in! The skin is a protective shield. Any break in the skin is an opening through which blood flows out, and microorganisms and contaminates can enter.

Dental professionals should take great care before cleaning the mouth of a person with PI. This includes good oral hygiene instruction and nutritional supplements before any dental cleaning is done. If a serious PI condition cannot be brought under control then, in order to manage the infection, a course of antibiotics may be indicated.

However, there is growing controversy as to whether a person with a healthy mouth who has heart irregularities, such as mitral valve prolapse, should be pre-medicated with an antibiotic before dental treatment to prevent the infection called subacute bacterial endocarditis (SBE). The theory is that SBE is caused by oral bacteria traveling in the bloodstream and adhering to damaged heart valves.

The first premise is that during dental treatment bacteria are dislodged from their hiding places and travel through the blood vessels (bacteremia). *This is true only if there are bacteria in the mouth to dislodge.*

The second premise is that an antibiotic administered one-hour before any dental treatment will kill any bacteria in the bloodstream. The antibiotic of choice is amoxicillin.

However, almost 50% of the targeted microbes are now resistant to amoxicillin. Others point out that, since amoxicillin never eliminates the bacteria completely, its routine administration could lead to the creation of more super-bugs.[137,138,139,139,140]

The third premise is that, in a mouth with PI, the possibility of a bacteremia resulting in SBE is always present. Brushing, flossing or even chewing can cause bleeding. *What bleeds out, bleeds in.*[141]

The fourth premise is that many people postpone going to the dentist to avoid taking antibiotics that have previously made them ill. *By putting off dental visits, the chance of developing PI may be increased. This delay could set the stage for a bacteremia.*

Why bother giving a questionable treatment that sometimes carries severe side effects and adverse reactions? If a healthy mouth has few or no bugs, then there are few bugs to invade the circulatory system. This approach requires an enthusiastic individual and a cooperative dental team. Maintaining a healthy mouth improves overall health, is gentle on the immune system, and will not encourage antibiotic resistance.

To protect against subacute bacterial endocarditis the answer is not to take antibiotics before dental visits but to eliminate PI.

Tetracycline

The use of long-term, low-dose tetracycline has recently been shown to improve PI. One of its methods of action is to inhibit the destructive inflammatory enzyme, collagenase. There are natural ways to inhibit this enzyme without encouraging antibiotic resistance to the antibiotic. These alternative approaches will be discussed later in the book.[142]

Antacids

You may want to rethink taking antacids. During the 1970s, histamine blockers were created to help with indigestion. These drugs, including Zantac, Pepcid AC and Tagamet, along with antacids like Tums and Rolaids, were designed to stop or greatly reduce hydrochloric acid (HCL) in the stomach. *However, from our microbiological understanding, HCL destroys the bacteria that we ingest every time we eat or drink. It is one of the body's first lines of defense. Without HCL, we automatically allow bad bacteria to enter into our bodies.*[143]

What You Can Do

Just say no to antibiotics! Most periodontal problems can be successfully treated without the use of antibiotics.[144,145] If specific circumstances warrant the use of an antibiotic, it should only be administered by your dentist after a culture is analyzed to determine the appropriate antibiotic to use.[146]

Diagnosing Periodontal Infection

Reality: No One Wants To Go To The Dentist!

Have you ever heard anyone say, "Wow, today I'm going to the dentist, and I'm so excited!" I don't think so. With the recognition of PI as a health hazard, however, people will realize they can increase the probability of living longer, healthier lives if they take care of their dental problems. They will also appreciate that combining a sound, home oral health initiative with a program of professional care will benefit not only their appearance but their overall health.

Diagnosing PI Without A Dental Visit

Any oral discomfort or abnormal coloring can indicate infection. Unfortunately from a detection point of view, gum disease isn't associated with a great deal of pain, especially in its early phases. Without pain, the majority of people aren't adequately concerned about their teeth and gums.

You can keep a sharp lookout for PI by being aware of the following symptoms:

- **Bleeding** is the most common marker of infection. Small ulcers or wounds in the gum pocket bleed with the smallest provocation, such as flossing, brushing, irrigating, or even rinsing and chewing. If you see even a little blood when you are cleaning your mouth, there is a problem!

- **Red, swollen or tender gums** are an indication of PI.

- **Abscesses** are swellings or bumps on the gum surface that can either appear suddenly or grow gradually. They can feel hot and/or painful. An abscess always indicates PI.

- **Discomfort** resulting from inflammation as pressure is exerted on the nerves. Note carefully which teeth are sensitive to pain and whether this condition is constant or fluctuates. If the area is irrigated with an anti-microbial and the discomfort goes away, the source for the pain is most likely PI. However, if the discomfort is a throbbing pain, and cold relieves it, the infection is probably into the nerve, and the tooth needs immediate attention.

- **Gums** that have pulled away from the teeth are a clear indication of PI.

- **Loose, shifting teeth,** or a change in the way teeth or partial dentures fit together when you bite, is an indication of PI.

- **Persistent bad breath** is usually caused by hydrogen sulfide compounds, which are bacterial waste products. It is almost always a sign of PI. One way to determine if the cause is PI is to floss and then smell the floss. If it smells bad, like rotten eggs or spoiled food, PI is probably present.

- **Medications** can also cause bleeding. Anti-convulsants (dilantin) or hypertensive drugs like the calcium channel blockers (Cardizem, Tenormin) can cause hyperplasia,

---

The Periodontal Coyote

The coyote—or trickster—in Indian folklore represents something that is not as it seems. In PI, sometimes the gum line remains stable, but the bone starts receding away, giving the illusion that there is no problem. Unfortunately, this happens with good brushers who rarely visit the dentist and have no idea of what's happening below the gum line.

---

abnormal overgrowth of gum tissue. Aspirin and most anticoagulant medicines will also cause a patient to bleed more easily.

- **Dental plaque** is hard to see. Chewing red disclosing tablets, sold at grocery stores and drug stores, can stain plaque, making it more visible. Another technique to make plaque visible is to paint red food coloring on the teeth after brushing. The color left on the teeth shows where there is still plaque.

The Fantasy of Relying on Home Care

Tooth product manufacturers convey the message that their products will help you to avoid going to the dentist for regular cleanings and dental check-ups. Unfortunately, most dental challenges are not apparent until the situation is serious. The truth is that, even if you have healthy looking gums, until a dentist examines your dental state, you have no proof whether or not microscopic pathogens have adopted your gums as home sweet home.

Diagnosing PI at the Dental Office

Most people rely on their dentist to take responsibility for their teeth. From a young age we are told to visit the dentist every six months. We assume that if something is wrong with our teeth or gums, the dentist will find it. Based on the abysmal PI statistics, the six-month recall is generally inadequate and scientifically unfounded.

As a note of interest, a famous television commercial informed everyone in the 1950's to brush their teeth and visit their dentist every six months. Insurance companies adopted this visitation regime when dental insurance was made available to the public.

To prevent and control PI, a rigorous program must be maintained. If an active periodontal infection is present, visiting the dentist four times or more a year is highly recommended, and following a biological oral hygiene system at home is a must.[148]

Procedures

Most dentists consider beginning gingivitis, at worst, a low-grade infection without serious consequences. As a matter of fact, many dental professionals view gum disease as a minor problem affecting everyone as they age. Unfortunately, if PI is not acted on early enough, gum surgery or extraction will be needed.

Even as gum infection is spreading and perhaps developing into oozing pockets of bacteria-laden pus, it still may go unnoticed. Can you imagine ignoring any other infection that is spreading down to the bone and possibly destroying the bone itself? Probably not, yet this is exactly what is happening in a mouth with gum disease.

X-Rays

The most common diagnostic device used is the **x-ray**. This tool gives the dentist a better understanding of the dental situation, including the location of small cavities, contours of the bone supporting the teeth, the thickness and shape of the periodontal ligament, gum development and deposits of calculus at the gum line.

In its early stages, PI does not have many overt signs detectable by x-ray but as it progresses, the body reabsorbs the bone around the teeth, causing bone loss. Identification of beginning bone loss with an x-ray is essential to early rectification of a PI problem.

Moderation is the most important rule to follow regarding x-ray exposure. A full set of around eighteen small x-rays should not be repeated more than every three to five years.

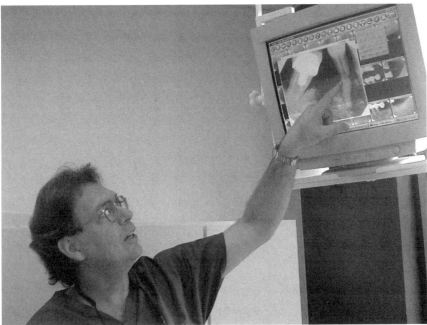

New digital x-ray technology - *reduces patient exposure to radiation by 90% and significantly enhances a dentist's ability to diagnose PI.*

However, new digital x-ray equipment represents a break-through in technology because the patient is exposed to 90% less radiation. This kind of x-ray uses a sensor and computer instead of film. The benefits are:

- Immediately viewable

- Able to measure more accurately the level of bone loss and to locate deposits of calculus

- Easily enlarged in questionable areas

- Able to enhance images by changing the contrast and color to aid in early detection of problems

- Capable of recording short-term changes in bone structure; minute changes in bone formation can be detected in as little as four months

- Available on a diskette that can be stored in the patient's file in the office, on the patient's computer, or e-mailed to another specialist

- Less chemical vapors in the dental office and pollution from x-ray processing

Caution: During any X-ray exposure, be sure your dentist protects you with a lead apron that also surrounds the neck.

I suggest taking a copy of your x-rays home, either on a diskette to save on your own computer or printed. Comparing older x-rays with newer ones is very useful.

The panoramic x-ray allows viewing of the whole mouth at once. Put in geographical terms, it is like seeing the entire Grand Canyon all at once, as opposed to just a cliff at a time. Problem areas, such as the jaw joint, shape of the jaw, bone

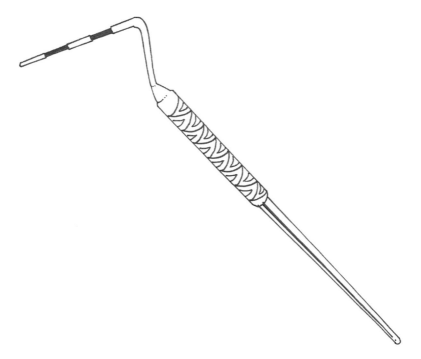

Periodontal Probe - *Its end is marked to measure pocket depth in millimeters.*

levels around teeth, areas of inflammation, sinuses, and even the carotid artery, are visible.

Probing & Charting

A periodontal exam continues with **charting** the contours of the gums and pocket depths. This is accomplished by the use of an instrument called the perio-probe. The probe is like a small ruler marked off in millimeters that can be inserted into the gingival crevice. Six readings are taken around each tooth, and the presence or absence of bleeding is recorded.

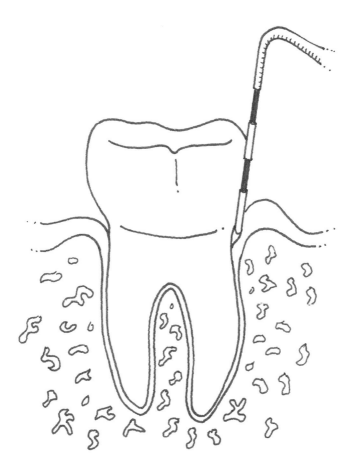

A periodontal probe in a healthy sulcus measures 2mm depth.

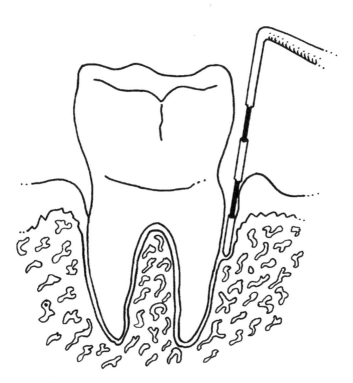

A periodontal probe in a pocket with moderate PI measures 6mm in depth.

The recording is used as a long-term gauge to determine if PI has been eliminated or is still a problem.

Many dentists rely on **probing** to determine periodontal condition. Probing only measures previous disease progression and cannot tell if infection is currently present. Bleeding usually indicates trouble but, as noted earlier, prescription drugs can affect this condition.

The mobility of each tooth should be determined. Teeth that make contact improperly may become loose, wear unevenly, be sensitive to temperature changes, or become painful. Mobility can also be caused by bone loss. In any of the above situations, an irritated tooth that is loose is susceptible to bacteria entering the periodontal ligament.

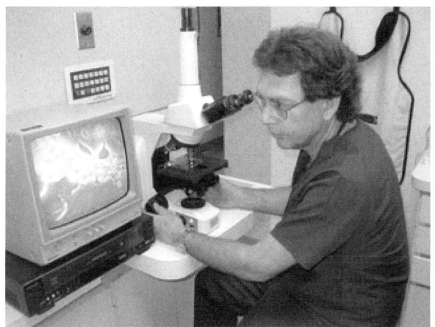

The author seated at a phase-contrast microscope, viewing bugs from a patient's mouth.

Phase-Contrast Microscopy

The best tool a dentist can have in the war against bugs is a **phase-contrast video microscope** (source: OraTec.com). It makes the invisible visible, allowing the viewer to see live parasites, bacteria, protozoa and fungus that live between the teeth and gums. The procedure requires a sample of plaque from the bottom of the deepest pockets. This plaque is placed on a slide and then examined under the microscope.

The plaque—and whatever lives in it—is seen on a monitor connected to the microscope. At this point, bugs are enlarged to 1000 times their actual size. The viewer can easily see the microorganisms and determine their level of activity and concentration. This procedure is quick, painless, easy, and can show the seriousness of the infection.

The phase-contrast microscope can rapidly identify white blood cells (WBCs). Since increases in WBCs are determined by the host's immune system, their presence provides strong

---

Classes of Risk Factors

Phase Contrast Microscope at 1000x magnification

Class 1 is more than 10 white blood cells (WBCs), low numbers of spinning rods, spiraling rods and gliding rods.

Class 2 is more than 50 WBCs, much more movement, a few spirochetes, and less than 25 cigar shaped rods.

Class 3 WBCs may be greater than 50 per field, and the area is alive with movement. Counting specific pathogens may be almost impossible. Spirochetes are dominating and starting to organize, especially around WBCs.

Class 4 sees banks of WBCs and much larger spirochetes that are organized and swimming in well-defined waves. Large cigar rods and protozoa (amoebas and trichemonas) are common. The screen is covered with pathogenic life.

---

evidence of ongoing inflammation and infection. WBCs are usually present long before periodontal destruction is noticeable.

In addition to its ability to assess periodontal microflora, the microscope is an extremely effective motivator. While patients may realize that plaque is composed of bacteria, actually seeing their own living bugs on a video monitor is a dramatic experience that usually results in significantly improved home care.

Testing

Genetic tests are available to assess the presence of specific genes. In individuals with certain gene patterns, susceptibility to PI is much greater. In the future, preliminary laboratory tests may be routinely done by all dentists to prevent PI from ever occurring in those with these genetic configurations. For the present, however, there is a laboratory finger-stick test with one drop of blood that can be done by your dentist. If in-office treatment and at-home compliance is good, and PI persists, genetic vulnerability should become a suspect.[149,150,151]

Bacterial Culturing is done in specialized oral microbiology labs that culture and identify fifteen periodontal pathogens. Once a bug is identified, these labs provide a recommendation on the appropriate antibiotic to use. Culturing is the most sophisticated test currently available. The test requires several weeks to obtain results, and the specimen must be shipped overnight. If your dentist does not have a microscope, request a culture.[152]

The DNA probe is the most sensitive test and is usually done at the same lab that is doing the culture. These labs use DNA probes to detect organisms like spirochetes that cannot be cultured. DNA probes only test for a limited number of species, typically three to seven, to determine the presence of pathogenic organisms that may not have grown out in the culture but were present in the sample. Such anaerobes may be difficult to grow outside of the mouth but are readily identified by their genetic remnants (the footprint of a bug).

An important feature of this test is that the anaerobes do not have to be alive. Test results reflect the presence of, and approximate number of, tested pathogens. This type of DNA test is similar to the test performed in criminal investigations, which looks for species-specific sequences of bacteria. Since the bacteria are no longer alive, DNA probes, unlike cultures, cannot provide antibiotic specificity data.

The **BANA (benzoyl-DL-arginine-naphthylamide) test,** developed by Dr. Walter Loesche of the University of Michigan, detects microbes that are associated with PI. The BANA test identifies the bacteria *P. gingivalis*, *B. forsythus* and

T. denticola. These three species possess an enzyme that is capable of hydrolyzing BANA. Plaque samples are taken from four sites; if three of the four test positive, PI is present. This test does not take the place of a microscope or a laboratory culture, but it is quick, easy and inexpensive. It is done in the dental office.[153,154]

The **2000 Probe** measures small levels of hydrogen sulfide gas released by bacteria. The new rapid-screening 2000 Probe produces immediate results in the dental office.

The **Halimeter** is generally associated with testing for halitosis (bad breath) by measuring hydrogen sulfides. Sulfide production is largely a by-product of anaerobic bacteria. High hydrogen sulfide levels suggest the presence of bacteria. Most bad-breath originates from the anaerobes living in the coating on the back of the tongue.

A Description of the Enemy

Pathogenic microorganisms tend to be mobile: increased mobility often correlates to increased virulence.

Bacteria

- **Spirochetes** look like snakes. With their constant spiraling motion, they worm their way into the tissue of the gum. They can eat right through the skin to feast on blood and fibrin. If your gums bleed easily, always suspect the presence of spirochetes.

- **Small gliding rods** are short, cigar-looking bugs that cruise rapidly from one end of the screen to the other. They are fairly tough to kill. They may grow on bone and eventually destroy it.

- **Large gliding rods** are long and graceful. They also may destroy bone.

- **Spinning rods** are the whirling dervishes of the bug world. They are very active, constantly twirling. Unfortunately, these colorful bugs are associated with progressive PI.

- **Clock Arms (Cytophaga)** look like they were designed to tell the time, with extended, pole-like arms swinging like the hands of a clock.

- **Motile cocci** are small specks that zip around the slide. Sometimes these bugs are seen in the slides of children who do not brush carefully enough. They can cause bleeding and mild irritation.

One-Celled Animals

- **Trichomonas tenax** look like miniature mice with five extended tentacles flailing in front as they overcome any bacteria in their way.

- **Amoebas** are shapeless blobs that creep about in slow motion. Their shape depends on what they have just eaten. They devour white blood cells after first stinging them. When a white blood cell is stung, it goes in to frenzy, releasing enzymes that dissolve the surrounding tissue. This degrading of the tissue calls for even more white blood cells, which meet a similar fate. Since amoebas are asexual and are capable of reproducing quickly, the increase in damaged white blood cells provides more food for the ever-growing amoeba colony. They alone may do more damage than any other microorganism.

- **Yeast, fungus and candida** are slow moving and are either long strands, which are invasive, or dots that can grow rapidly. This pathogen has the capability of switching functions, depending on which stage it is in.

Periodontal Care in the Dental Office

Your dentist has excellent ways to fight gum disease. In addition, if your general dentist does not specifically treat gum problems, he will refer you to a periodontist. A periodontist has had three years of advanced training in the treatment of PI and other oral health problems.

The most common treatment in either office is the prophylaxis, or cleaning. The dental hygienist, an integral member of either dental team, normally cleans teeth. Even if you are an ardent tooth brusher and flosser, there may be places you routinely miss. The hygienist will clean these areas, show you how to improve your home care, and coach you through any learning process. This is a good opportunity to bring in devices, such as your electric toothbrush or irrigator, for hands-on instruction.

Plaque is a sticky, colorless film that constantly forms on your teeth. If plaque is not removed, it hardens into a rough, porous deposit called *calculus*, or *tartar*. This deposit is similar in structure to a miniature coral reef and makes a protected shelter for many pathogens. Microorganisms and their toxic by-products irritate the gums and make them red, tender, swollen and more likely to bleed. As this build-up continues, it can destroy supporting gum tissue around teeth, forming pockets that fill with more plaque. When this condition is ignored, the bone supporting the tooth can be damaged.

Deep pocket cleanings are procedures called *curettage*, *scaling* and *root planing*. These steps are performed when a regular cleaning is no longer effective. These non-surgical techniques are done well below the gum line.

Curettage is the thorough cleaning of the soft tissue lining the pocket. **Scaling** removes deposits of bacterial plaque, calculus, food debris and pus that have accumulated in the infected pocket. **Root planing** smoothes and cleans the root of the tooth, so that the gum tissue may heal next to the tooth.

Together, they are designed to remove calculus, which is attached to cementum, the protective shield of the root. It is important to remove as little cementum as possible because taking away cementum can expose the porous dentin of the root to microbial invasion.[155,156] Removing just the right amount of hardened calculus and plaque under the gums will allow the gum area to heal and reattach. Deep cleaning requires an instrument called an *ultrasonic* or *piezo scaler* that dislodges calculus and flushes away debris with a stream of antimicrobial solution. This action simultaneously cleans and disinfects the pocket.

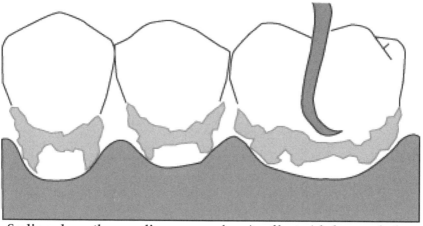

Scaling above the gum line *removes deposits of bacterial plaque, calculus, food debris and pus.*

Deep cleaning is a beneficial step in controlling PI. Although it sounds complicated, it is a non-traumatic course of action, with little post-op discomfort. In most cases, deep cleaning requires anesthesia.

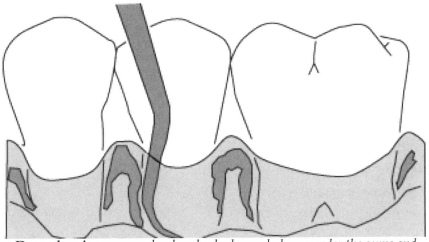

Deep cleaning *removes hardened calculus and plaque under the gums and allows the gum area to heal and reattach.*

Sometimes a deep cleaning cannot reach an infected root area that is hidden beneath the curtain of the gum. These cases may require surgery, which allows the dentist to visibly see and correct the areas that are not responding to more conservative treatments. Surgery removes hidden calculus and inflamed tissue from deep pockets. In a procedure referred to as a *gingivectomy*, excessive gum tissue is trimmed to reduce pocket size.

Periodontal surgery also smoothes root surfaces and arranges gum tissue into a shape that will be easier to keep clean. Modern equipment, local anesthesia and new techniques make this treatment more comfortable than it used to be. Today, it is mildly painful for a day or two and requires about eight weeks to fully heal.

Two other procedures that are performed in a periodontist office to help the PI patient are *gingival* or *soft tissue grafts* and *osseous surgery.*

Gingival grafts are designed to replace or enhance the amount of gum supporting a tooth. When there is inadequate gum remaining to support a tooth, or excessive recession exposes the root, PI quite often develops. When this happens, these areas can be covered with a graft of new gum tissue often taken from another part of the mouth. Cosmetically, this can eliminate the "long-in-the-tooth" look which, for some, denotes an aging appearance. A reverse of this procedure is used when infection causes the gums to grow excessively and become puffy, creating a "gummy smile."

Osseous surgery is designed to modify and reshape the bone surrounding the tooth. This is a necessary procedure in the effective treatment of advanced PI because uneven progression of the disease causes an odd configuration of bony support. New materials of either artificial or freeze-dried bone can fill in for lost bone.

Great Oral Health

Home Care Hygiene Techniques

Brushing is inexpensive and very effective. Use a soft bristle toothbrush that bends and conforms to the surface of your teeth. Toothbrush size depends on the size of the mouth. For example, small mouths require small toothbrushes. When in doubt use a small brush, just because it is easier to maneuver in the mouth.

The most important part of brushing is to make sure that every tooth gets clean. Being thorough is more important than brushing hard. The British Dental Health Foundation said regular brushing can miss up to 40% of the food particles in the mouth.[157]

Brush at least once a day; two or more times are better. If brushing is not possible, rinse thoroughly with water. This is especially important if sugar is consumed.

If possible, brush after each meal. Plaque reorganizes and colonizes every twenty-four hours, so it is important to prevent this from happening.

Thorough brushing should take three to five minutes. A quick once-over can be done in less than thirty seconds and will remove some food debris. But do not be fooled, you have not cleaned your teeth.

Inappropriate brushing, especially horizontal tooth brushing, is a common cause of gingival recession and tooth-surface abrasion. Many types of toothpaste are too abrasive.[158] Although they clean quickly, they are like scraping your teeth with sand. . To avoid tooth erosion choose a toothpaste that is gentle on the tooth surface and highly effective against PI.

It is very easy to become re-infected with a bacteria-laden toothbrush! Bugs thrive in cool, dark humid spaces, just the type of place people like to store their toothbrushes. A pair of moist toothbrushes left side by side in the bathroom medicine cabinet can definitely make a PI exchange.[159]

If an active infection is present, toothbrushes must be replaced at least every two weeks. Also, toothbrushes should be replaced after you or your family members have had any upper respiratory tract infection, such as the flu or a cold.[160,161,162,163,164]

> *Toothbrushes kept in a moist environment like that of a bathroom retained up to 50% of herpes simplex virus Type I for a week.[167]*

Toothbrushes can be replaced or sterilized with full strength hydrogen peroxide for at least thirty minutes or, for better sanitation, they can be stored in hydrogen peroxide. They can also be stored in a mouthwash solution containing essential oils, which kill 100% of the bacteria present. Both solutions should be replaced daily. The use of a UV sanitizing device also has shown to be effective.[165,166]

Always use a soft toothbrush. Toothbrushes labeled anything other than soft are too rough and may loosen the bond between gum tissue and the tooth.

> *In a recent article, the Journal of the American Dental Association (JADA) suggested that dental professionals advise their patients who have PI to disinfect or change their toothbrushes between brushings to prevent self-infection.[168]*

Some pointers:

- Angle the bristles of the brush along the gum line at a 45-degree angle. Most of the plaque that is missed in a "quickie" brushing is at the gum line and between the teeth.

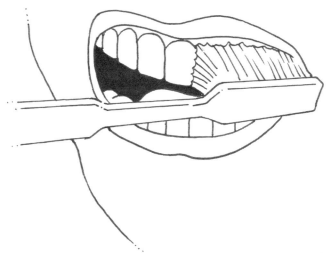

To clean the outer surfaces of the teeth, keep the brush at a 45° angle to the teeth. Focus on touching the gums, and gently move the brush back and forth using short strokes. End by brushing away from the gums.

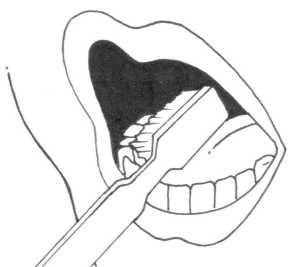

Brush the inside surfaces in the same way as the outer surfaces. Keep contact with the gums.

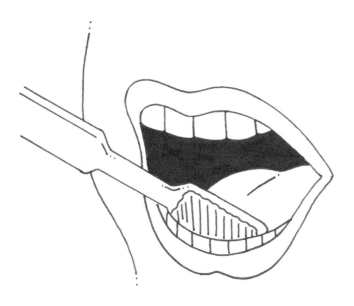

Behind the lower front teeth is an area that builds calculus easily. Use the tip of the brush to scrub this surface vigorously.

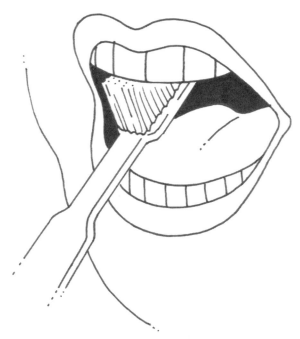

The inner surface of the upper front teeth is cleaned by holding the brush vertically and using and up and down motion.

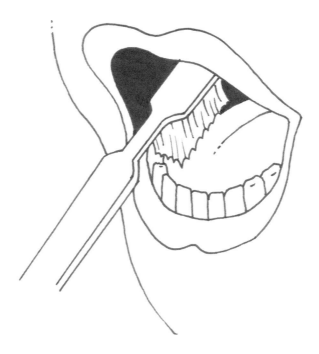

The chewing surfaces of the back teeth are cleaned with an in-and-out stroke.

■ Apply firm pressure so that the bristles slide under the gum line.

■ Vibrate the brush while it is moved in short back and forth strokes and in small circular motions.

■ Brush two or three teeth at a time, then move to the next teeth, allowing some overlap.

■ Tilt the brush and use the tip to brush the backs of the front teeth.

■ It is fine to brush in any regular pattern a person may choose but, since the insides of the teeth tend to get less attention, a person might start with the insides of the upper teeth, then to the insides of the lower teeth.

- Switch to the outside of the upper teeth, and then the outside of the lower teeth.

- Brush the chewing surfaces of the upper teeth, then the lower teeth.

- End by gently brushing the tongue (see tongue scraping) and the roof of the mouth.

Dry brushing without any toothpaste or wetting compound is also effective against plaque build up. A soft toothbrush is used to scour away built-up bacterial plaque with the inner surfaces of the bottom row of teeth brushed first, before saliva buildup develops. Proceed to the inner top level of teeth next, and then move to the outer surface.

For added benefit, place a drop of an anti-microbial solution or gel on a toothbrush and brush around the gum tissue, with the bristles of the toothbrush angled toward the gums. Work the gel up under the tissue as much as possible. Leave the anti-microbial on the tissue. Do not rinse or wipe it off.

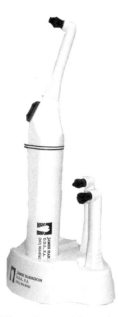

An electric toothbrush may be more effective at plaque control and cause less risk of trauma to gingival tissue than a manual toothbrush. The head of this electric brush should be small and round, allowing the brush to clean one tooth at a time. It uses very soft bristles that come to a small point. The brush turns slowly and causes minimal abrasion. Only one to two seconds per tooth is required.

The soft bristles gently massage the junction where the tooth meets the gum. This is not an aggressive action. No harm will be done to the most delicate tissue, and even the places where erosion is pres-

Electric toothbrush

ent will be cleaned. If you like the way your teeth feel after a visit to the hygienist, then using the right electric brush will give you a similar feeling.[169,170,171]

Do not use toothpaste with an electric brush. Toothpastes formulated for hand brushing are too abrasive to use with an electric brush. However, an anti-microbial solution or gel can be used to moisten, deodorize, and add an anti-bug cleaning effect.

Rinse with an anti-microbial mouthwash. Vigorously rinse or swish for 30 to 60 seconds, expectorate the excess and do not rinse with water. For superior results, refrain from eating or drinking for 15 to 30 minutes.

Prescription and over-the-counter mouth rinses often contain a considerable amount of alcohol. In addition to alcohol, these products have other ingredients, such as detergents, emulsifiers, organic acids and azo dyes. These are harmful additives that are easily absorbed through the mucosa lining of the mouth, and may cause cancer.[172]

Flossing or using toothpicks can disrupt, loosen and remove plaque that cannot be reached with brushing. Flossing cleans the area between the teeth, but not in deep pockets. Flossing helps to control PI.[173,174]

Floss at least once a day. The best time to floss is after the last food of the day. Floss in front of a mirror until you become proficient. If you are unable to floss due to an injury or an illness, there are mechanical devices available. Waterpik® makes a good electric flosser. Also, if you can't get the floss between two teeth, use a floss threader.

Several types of floss or dental tape are available. Unwaxed floss is thinner than waxed and is best for getting into tight areas; however,

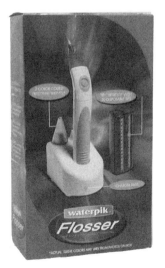

Electric flosser

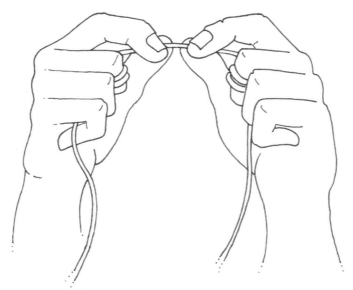

Using about 18 inches of floss, wrap most around one middle finger. Wrap the rest around the other middle finger. Holding the floss between the thumbs and forefinger, gently slide the floss between the teeth.

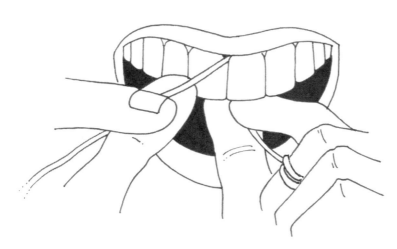

Gently slide the floss between the teeth. Try not to pop it through tight contacts. Going beneath the gums is not recommended.

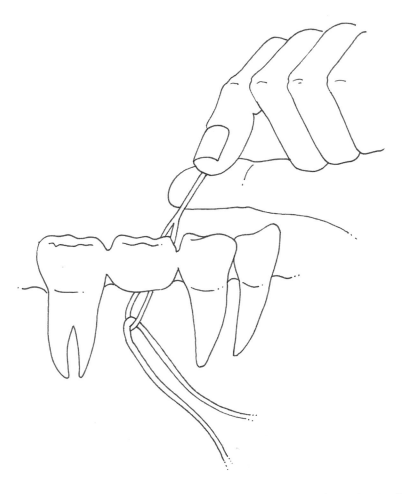

Using a floss threader or a floss with a molded-in threader will greatly simplify cleaning under a bridge.

unwaxed floss frays more easily. Unwaxed is the best for removing plaque. Waxed floss is easier if rough areas are present or teeth are close together. If you want to use unwaxed and have problem areas where the floss gets stuck or shreds, you may want to try one of the newer brands designed to slide between the teeth. (However, if floss continues to shred this is an indication to see you dentist to have rough and tight areas checked.) If the floss becomes red from bleeding, don't stop! Bleeding is a sign that you have PI, and your gums need extra attention.

A few pointers:

- Floss is inexpensive. A new section should be used for each tooth. Pay special attention if the floss turns red from bleeding.

- Wind eighteen inches of dental floss around the middle fingers of each hand, leaving about five inches between the hands.

- Pinch the floss between the thumbs and index fingers and leave about one inch in-between to work with.

- Use a sawing motion, gently bringing the floss through the tight spaces of the teeth.

- If the teeth are too tight to floss, or if the floss catches or tears, the dentist should be notified.

- Pull the floss tightly in a C shape around the side of the tooth and slide it under the gum line.

- Do not snap the floss against the gums.

- Curve the floss around each tooth and gently scrape from just below the gum to the top of the tooth several times.

- Never force dental floss deep into the gums.

- When all the plaque has been removed, you will hear the floss start to squeak.

- Wind the floss to a fresh section.

- Always rinse or irrigate after flossing, preferably with an antimicrobial solution.
  Caution: A taught strand of dental floss can cut your gums like a piano-wire cuts cheese. Be gentle.

Interproximal brushes look like a pipe cleaner with a small-rounded brush on the end. These brushes can reach back teeth, and the smallest ones can be used for pocket cleansing. To enhance effectiveness they can be dipped into an anti-microbial solution or gel.

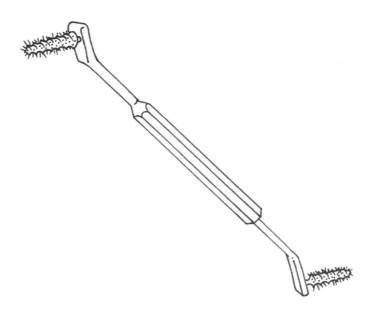

Interproximal Brushes

Tongue-scraping. 75% of mouth odors (halitosis) come from the tongue. It is also the main breeding area for anaerobic bacteria that live under the coating on the tongue. Eliminating this coating exposes the bacteria to oxygen and also removes a great quantity of debris.

Cleaning the tongue reduces overall dental plaque on the teeth by 33%. If the tongue is not scraped, bacteria recolonize the teeth after brushing. To prevent re-infection of treated periodontal sites, all areas of the oral cavity must be clean.[175,176]

To improve the effectiveness of tongue cleaning, apply an anti-microbial before scraping the tongue. This not only removes the coating, but also helps to kill any remaining bugs.

Irrigating is an excellent technique for controlling PI. Mouth rinsing reaches about 0.2 millimeters below the gums, and tooth brushing reaches 0.9 millimeters. Irrigation can reach more than six millimeters deep. Irrigation washes away food particles and plaque below the gum line. More importantly, it is an excellent way to deliver antimicrobial solutions.[177,178]

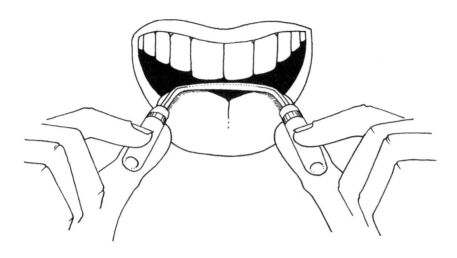

Most breath mal-odor comes from the back of the tongue. Place the tongue scraper as far back on the tongue as possible and gently pull forward. Rinse the scraper and repeat until the tongue is clean.

There are two types of irrigation:

1. *Supragingival irrigation* works above the gum line. Several studies show that supraginigival irrigation provides benefits beyond that of tooth brushing for controlling plaque. This occurs because the irrigators flush out bacteria and project water or antimicrobial solutions up to 3 millimeters below the gum line.[179,180]

2. *Subgingival irrigation* is truly the at-home weapon for controlling PI. It works in pockets 6 or more millimeters deep. This type of irrigation requires a device with special applicator tips designed to reach below the gum line. These tips must be inserted carefully into the gingival crevice to direct the flow of antimicrobials so that the solution reaches the bottom of the pocket.[181,182]

Caution: Always use low to moderate pressure with any power irrigator. High pressure can damage delicate tissue.

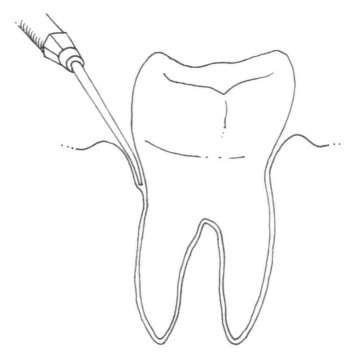

Irrigator with a thin tip easily reaches to the bottom of a pocket. Always use low to medium pressure.

Irrigating the whole mouth need not take longer than five minutes. The plaque below the gums is not sticky like the plaque above the gums. **The purpose of the irrigator is to distribute an antimicrobial agent deep to the bottom of the pocket, not to pressure clean the mouth**.

For most people irrigating is easier than flossing. It requires less dexterity, you don't need small fingers and you don't have to open your mouth as wide.

WaterPik® Professional model, Hydro Floss®, ViaJet® and other oral irrigators offer attachments for subgingival irrigation. Some offer a smaller tub that holds around 10 ounces (300 cc) of

The best time for your oral hygiene program is just before bed-time, because this provides the cleanest mouth for the longest period of time. However, if your are too fatigued by bedtime then do the full program after dinner and a "quickie" before bed.

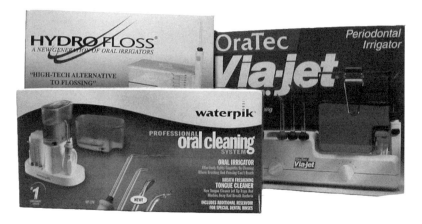

Irrigators - *above are three models which are very effective for home use.*

liquid, which is enough to thoroughly distribute solution to all areas of the mouth without wasting the anti-microbial. New to the market are a portable electric irrigator from Panasonic® and a convenient squeeze-bottle pocket irrigator from OraTec® (oratec.net).

Therapeutics for Oral Irrigation Devices

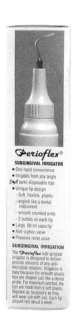

The ideal irrigating solution combines antimicrobials, connective tissue rebuilders and tissue conditioners to create an unfriendly environment for a wide variety of microorganisms. It does not just suppress their activity, but it enhances the host's resistance. The ingredients should be natural, non-toxic and supported by valid claims and research. The next chapter provides information about natural products that are commercially available for therapeutic, maintenance or preventative purposes.

Solutions other than commercially available natural antimicrobials can also be useful in

Portable Irrigators - *Portable irrigators like the one at the left are perfect for travel or other use outside the home.*

combating PI. Each has positive and negative features. The following recipes are based on using 10 ounces (300 cc) of warm potable water with the ingredient described below. If the oral irrigator you choose is different in size, calculate the difference.

1. Plain water can reduce microflora; use it, if nothing else is available.[183]

2. Two teaspoons of baking soda (sodium bicarbonate) is a salt that is four times more bactericidal than regular table salt. Because undissolved crystals are bad for the machine, it is best to mix the powder in a glass container and then add the solution to the irrigator tub. Thoroughly rinse the irrigator after use. Unless considerable amounts of the mixture are swallowed, no significant amount of sodium is absorbed through the oral mucosa, making it safe for those on salt restricted diets.

3. One teaspoon of table salt (sodium chloride) can dehydrate microorganisms. Unfortunately it can also dehydrate the teeth, causing sensitivity for a short period. Caution: only use an irrigator marked "safe for salt." Because undissolved crystals are bad for the machine, it is best to mix the powder in a glass container and then add the solution to the irrigator tub. Always thoroughly rinse the irrigator after use. Unless considerable amounts of the mixture are swallowed, the amount of sodium chloride absorbed through the oral mucosa is insignificant.

4. Three capfuls of 3% hydrogen peroxide diluted in ten ounces (300 cc) of water is a potent antimicrobial. It is the substance that our defensive cells release to kill invaders. However, peroxide is destructive to the connective tissue that supports the teeth. It can be used occasionally, but should not be used on a regular basis.

5. One-half teaspoon of bleach (sodium hypchlorite) is an effective killer of bugs; however, it is a chemical and is toxic.

Bleach is caustic, tastes terrible and is poisonous if swallowed.

6. Three and one-half ounces of vinegar acidifies the mouth, creating an unfriendly environment for bugs. However, due to its low pH, it can dissolve teeth if used on a regular basis.

7. Ten percent povidone iodine diluted 50/50 with warm water is quite an effective antimicrobial; however, it tastes terrible, and stains teeth and anything else it touches.

8. TheraSol® is a powerful antimicrobial using two synergistic proprietary active agents, amphoteric quaternary surfactants. This product does not stain the teeth and has a pleasant taste.

9. Peridex® and Periogard® (0.2% chlorexidine, CHX) is probably the best-known antimicrobial in the dental profession because it has been researched for thirty years. Although it is an effective antimicrobial, it has considerable side effects. If used on a regular basis, it produces dark brown stains on the teeth and increases calculus in about 40% of users. Also, it cannot be used in bleeding pockets because it binds with blood, preventing the solution from penetrating the pocket. CHX is available with a prescription only from pharmacies as a 5% concentrate. Use 1 ounce of concentrate per 25 ounces of warm water to make a .2% solution.

The above irrigating solutions generally have considerable downside problems: brown tooth staining, undesirable taste, poisonous in increased amounts, and difficulty and complications of proper mixing and measuring. Whether the limitations are one or several, most people give up too early in the treatment process to have any success. I generally recommend the commercially available natural products I discuss in the next chapter over any of the above solutions.

Children

Brushing a child's teeth is the same, whether done by an adult or the child. As soon as possible, a child should brush his or her own teeth to develop good oral hygiene habits. Most children, left to their own timing, will brush less than one minute. One to two minutes is the appropriate time, and a good way to reach that target is to use a timer. Some toothbrushes have clever timers that play music, so the child knows to finish when the music stops. Also, new battery-operated tooth bushes are like toys and, therefore, can amuse children when they are brushing. It is very important to check how effectively their cleaning is progressing. Coaching and demonstrating the appropriate technique is critical to the learning process.

The most important time to brush is before going to bed. This not only gives the bacteria less to feast on, but also addresses the condition of reduced saliva flow. Many of the same principles for adult brushing apply to children, such as brushing after sweets and, if that is not possible, then at least rinsing with water.

Again the techniques are similar to adult brushing and are the same whether an adult or the child does it. For small children, it may be easiest to cradle the head, leaving your other hand free for brushing.

Brushing

- Most beginning brushers tend to miss the molars and the tongue sides of the teeth.

- Place the toothbrush alongside the teeth. The bristle should be at a 45-degree angle.

- Carefully brush in a small circular motion, cleaning one tooth at a time, and being careful not to miss any teeth.

■ Brush across the chewing surfaces, especially making sure the bristles reach the side of the teeth facing the tongue, and the inside of the top teeth.

■ Brush the tongue lightly to remove bacteria and keep the breath smelling fresh.

■ Assist the child in rinsing his or her mouth.

Flossing

Flossing should begin once any two teeth touch each other. Generally a child can begin successfully flossing in the eight- to nine-year-old range.

■ Take about eighteen inches of dental floss, and wrap one end around each of your middle fingers.

■ Using your thumbs and index fingers as guides, gently slide the floss between the teeth with a saw-like motion.

■ Once at the gum line, pull the floss tightly but gently and move it up and down against one tooth.

■ Pull the floss against the other tooth and repeat the motion.

■ Repeat this for all of the teeth. Be sure to floss the farthest sides of the back teeth.

Brushing twice a day, and flossing at night before bedtime is important. Good oral health habits can be taught. However, the most important hygiene principles are learned through good examples.

Natural Products for Healthy Gums

T here are two objectives in promoting great oral health. The first objective is to reinforce the path to prevention so PI never occurs. The second is to bring any periodontal infection under control and support the regeneration process. When addressing PI, it is not enough to just brush and floss; a sophisticated protocol must be followed. The program that will be discussed in this section includes using natural antimicrobials and targeted nutritional supplements.

Antimicrobial Products

Several lines of natural, professional strength, oral hygiene products are now available. These products effectively address the periodontal issues of concerned patients and dentists. (Unfortunately government agencies restrict the use of the word *antimicrobial* on natural product labels so you have to read between the lines. *Antimicrobial* is allowed only on pharmaceuticals.)

What to look for when selecting a natural antimicrobial product

Ingredients: Aloe Vera, Folic Acid, Calendula flower, Echinacea purpurea tops, Gota Kola extract, Chlorophyll, Phytoplenolin Extract, Chamomile flower, Blood root, Prickly Ash Bark, Green tea leaf, Oregano leaf, Peppermint Oil, Cinnamon bark, Eucalyptus leaf, Lavender Oil, Bio-Saponin Conc., Co-Enzyme Q-10, Olive Leaf Extract, Black walnut green hulls, Clove leaf, Thyme herb, Grapefruit Seed Extract and vegetable glycerin.

These herbs and essential oils are known to kill microorganisms, reduce inflammation and rebuild damaged tissue. They are generally recognized as effective in one or more of these areas and should be included in any product purchased. A complete description of each begins on page 95.

Characteristics:

- Tastes good
- Promotes fresh breath
- Long-lasting
- Heals and maintains the health of gum tissue
- Kills existing micro-organisms at effective potency levels

Look for products that are manufactured with the following assurances:

- 100% natural herbal ingredients (organically grown or responsibly wild-crafted to ensure high amounts of bioactive substances)
- Vegetarian-based, without animal-derived by-products
- Alcohol-, chemical- and solvent-free (solvents strip the herbs of vital constituents)
- No artificial sweeteners, azo dyes and propylene glycol
- No sodium lauryl or laureth sulfate or harmful oxide derivatives
- No animal testing

Types of Products Available

Natural antimicrobial toothpaste does more than clean teeth; it also kills microorganisms in shallow pockets. Always look for products that are low in abrasion ingredients, such as calcium carbonate, silica and sodium bicarbonate (baking soda). Sodium bicarbonate is also an effective plaque inhibitor.[184,185,186] Toothpaste should leave the teeth feeling cleaner, and looking whiter and brighter.[187,188]

Natural antimicrobial mouthwashes are powerful full-strength oral rinses formulated for daily home care. They have been designed to adhere to oral tissue longer than most commercial products. Mouthwashes can also be used undiluted in handheld syringes for pocket irrigation, or as a toothpaste substitute with electric toothbrushes. Rinse for 30 to 60 seconds after brushing and flossing so there is enough time for the active ingredients to reach all areas of the mouth.

Natural antimicrobial irrigation solutions represent the foundation product in the war against PI. The solution creates an unfriendly environment that helps the body to expel the pathogens. Irrigation solutions must contain herbs and essential oils that are known for their anti-viral, anti-parasite and anti-fungal properties. They are formulated for patient and professional use in oral irrigation devices and are the ultimate weapon.

Natural antimicrobial balm or gel can be applied directly to the infected gum area. Gently massage the soothing balm into the gums around the infected teeth with a finger or cotton swab. Work the gel up under the tissue as much as possible. Antiseptic gels contain powerful ingredients; so a little amount provides a long-lasting, effective antimicrobial. This is an excellent product to use during the day, when traveling or away from an irrigator. Packaging in a tube allows for convenient dispensing of small amounts directly to a problem area. The potent ingredients in these products require just a small drop to not only kill bugs but also neutralize halitosis and freshen breath.

These antimicrobial products are available to control bugs and neutralize breath mal-odor, as well as fight cavities. Look for green tea extract, which is a powerful antioxidant. It also has been shown to inhibit the glue-forming enzyme that bacteria produce to attach themselves to tooth surfaces. In addition, green tea helps prevent plaque build-up and reduces decay.[189] Xylitol, a natural sweetener, has been shown to fight cavities and also remineralize tooth enamel.[190]

In the search for natural oral health products, folic acid is good because it increases absorption and enhances healing. Always look for natural botanical gum as the ingredient to thicken toothpaste, rather than a chemical formulation.[191]

Oral Nutrition

Several types of nutritional products that systemically address different aspects of PI treatment and prevention have been developed. Most of the products have unique for-mulations, allowing for enhanced absorption and bioavailability. The nutritional program chosen has to address the bacterial, viral and/or fungal challenges of the person with PI. The ingredients should be backed by scien-tific studies and clinical research.

The formulas should be recognized as phyto-nutrients; herbal extracts, selected co-enzymes, and specific vitamins and minerals, which strengthen and support the gums, teeth and immune system. These products, in combination with good oral hygiene, offer the potential to control PI, rebuild damaged tissue and, in many cases, prevent it from ever hap-pening.

Types of Products to Look For

There are four supplement formulations that are important for elimination, prevention and control of PI:

1. The **first formulation** helps to gain control over an active infection. This formulation will stop the release of bacterial enzymes and reduce the number of free radicals, which destroy gum tissue. Requirements for this formulation include: 1) stimulating the body's immune system and preventing bacteria from multiplying and going deeper into the gum tissue; 2) increasing ATP, the energy grid of the body, which also improves the healing response. The ingredients below encourage the development of healthy cells and should be included in any product you choose.

   Ingredients: Folic Acid, Vitamin B 12, Quercetin, Vitamin C, Vitamin A (from retinyl acetate), Echinacea, Grape Seed Extract, Co-enzyme Q10, Acetyl L-Carnitine, Selenium, Phytoplenolin, Olive Leaf, Black Pepper Extract

2. The **second formulation** provides a long-term shield against developing PI. It works by enhancing the biological resistance of the gums. Specific ingredients are included to bind the destructive proteins in the bacteria, inhibiting the development of PI.

   Ingredients: Vitamin E, Tocotrienols, Vitamin C with bioflavanoids and quercetins, Folic Acid, Vitamin B6, Vitamin B12, Selenium, Grape Seed Extract, Co-Enzyme Q10, Acetyl L-Carnitine, Alpha Lipoic Acid, Oleopein, Olive Leaf, Triphala, Black Pepper Extract

3. The **third formulation** is designed to promote bone remineralization. This type of nutritional supplement assists in restoring bone density.

   Ingredients: Calcium citrate and aspartate, Magnesium citrate and aspartate, Vitamin D3, Vitamin K, Vitamin

B6, Folic Acid, Vitamin B12, Biotin, Selenium (selenome-thionine), Boron (amino acid chelate), Manganese citrate, Copper gluconate, Zinc, Molybdenum, Silica (from oat straw and horsetail), Betaine HCL, Digestive plant enzymes, Grape Seed Extract, Silica, Triphala, Methionine, Black Pepper Extract

4. **The fourth formulation** is designed to be used together with any of the above formulations or taken alone. This formula provides a rich source of anti-oxidant protection and protection from the destructive collagen destroying enzymes released in inflammation. This will help control the spread of infection by stabilizing the connective tissue. Collagen building blocks are provided.

Ingredients: Vitamin C, Calcium, magnesium, Lysine, Proline and Vitamin B6.

Immediately after a dental visit

It is very important to prevent infection following an examination or dental procedure. Always rinse with an antiseptic solution before, during and after any treatment.

Take extra vitamin C for a couple of days after a dental procedure. If local anesthesia is given, vitamin C will help eliminate the after effects.

Caution: Do not take vitamin C in large doses before receiving local anesthesia because it may reduce the effectiveness of the anesthesia.

If your gums are overly sensitive following your dental visit, be more diligent and gentle during your dental routine. You may also want to massage a soothing balm into your gums.

The Periodontal Solutio

s I discussed in the first chapter, I began my quest to understand the causes and treatment of PI almost twenty years ago. The importance of this mission only increased as I uncovered research findings that linked this debilitating dental condition to even more serious health threats, such as heart disease.

As a pioneer in holistic dentistry, I like to think of myself as a leader in establishing new alternative standards. I became increasingly disturbed with the lack of available and effective periodontal products in the marketplace, even after major universities started releasing statistics correlating PI and life-threatening disease. This frustration led me to assist in developing several lines of natural products, sold and distributed here and abroad. My intent was that these products cover the full spectrum of a PI patient's dental needs—both for care in the dental office and care at home.

The nutritional company I have chosen to work with is Bio-Pro® Dental, a family-owned and operated company. Our philosophies are the same—produce the finest quality for the best results. Bio-Pro® Dental (866-924-6776) has been supplying nutritional-herbal products to the world for close to 30 years, about the same amount of time I have been addressing dental concerns.

Developing effective, good-tasting products that people will actually want to use was a challenge. I had to choose carefully from a wide variety of herbs and evaluate them for their ability to eliminate bugs without producing any undesirable side effects. Herbal extracts form the foundation of the products. Bio-Pro® Dental offers the only holistically-balanced herbal products on the market. These products had to keep the plant components in a state of natural wholeness, without adulterat-

Ancient healers understood and respected Mother Nature's intrinsic balance in plants and herbs. Herbalists have always appreciated that herbs are complex, comprised of thousands of chemical constituents working in synergy with each other. Traditional medicine is just beginning to understand this complexity.

ing naturally occurring bonds with toxic chemicals or solvents. The results are formulations that offer the maximum potential for healing.

Essential oils are an important component of each product. Oils represent the ethereal part of the plant. They are the subtle, volatile liquids distilled from flowers, bushes, trees, roots and even seeds. Oils are highly concentrated and much more potent than an individual herb. Sometimes, distillation of an entire plant may produce only one drop of oil. Essential oils' participation in healing has been woven into history from the beginning of time.

Their distinctive, lipid-soluble structure and minute size allow essential oils to easily penetrate cells and affect our immune system. The mosaic of an effective formula may be comprised of hundreds, if not thousands, of different chemicals. The knowledge required for each recipe is enormous. The average single oil may contain up to 200 chemical components, or even more, as seen with lavender. One chemical part of an essential oil may reduce inflammation, another may be antiseptic, and still another could have both properties.

Developing effective formulations was the first part of the challenge. Repeatedly and reliably producing them was the next hurdle.

The production process begins with the harvest. Each ingredient must be picked at the right time of day to insure maximum potency and the elimination of molds and fungus. After the correct choice of the right plants and oils by trained personnel, careful selection is made of the part to be processed—the flower, the leaves, seeds, stem, bark or roots.

Knowing how to handle each essential oil is important because they are delicate. Choosing the proper extraction method is critical. Efficiency is not an issue here, because quick methods with high temperatures and pressure processing will result in an inferior product.

Each step in the production process is crucial to producing exemplary results. Ultimately, this rigorous process culminates in transforming the herbs and oils into the final ingredients in a formulation.

I took great care in selecting quality manufacturing facilities. To my knowledge, Bio-Pro® Dental is the only herbal manufacturer with these credentials. Its facilities are custom-designed for the complex manufacture of herbal extracts and dietary supplements. They are state-of-art, and both FDA-registered and pharmaceutically licensed, guaranteeing the same quality, safety and scrutiny as in the prescription drug industry. They comply with cGMP (current Good Manufacturing Practices) and SOP (Standard Operating Procedures). Their in-house and microbiological testing laboratories observe GLP (Good Laboratory Practices), providing impeccable quality assurance.

The latest, most up-to-date list of sources can be found on my website, *www.theintegrativedentist.com*.

I hope you have found the information in this book helpful in understanding the serious consequences of untreated periodontal infection. More importantly, I hope you will use the tools and techniques I have described to protect your health and appearance.

And so this book comes to a close, but the journey continues. It's immensely gratifying—both personally and professionally—to hear from people who have achieved great oral health through natural means, so please consider this an open invitation to drop by the website and let me know how you are doing. I look forward to continuing the journey together.

Appendix A - Definitions

Acute infectious diseases are syndrome or illnesses that begin shortly after being exposed to an infection.

Alveolar bone is the bone that holds the teeth in place. The bone has different densities depending on the location in the mouth; the more strength required, the denser the bone. The body often reabsorbs (slowly removes) the bone if the

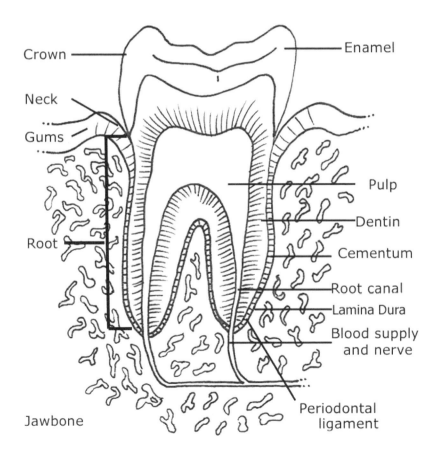

Anatomy of a tooth - *The diagram above shows a normal tooth and healthy gums.*

tooth is removed; leaving a depression in the gum after a tooth has been extracted.

Healthy bone on x-ray looks similar to sawdust and shows up with a pattern of lines of white surrounding dots of dark in a fairly uniform pattern. If the top edge of the bone between teeth has a thick white area at the surface, the bone is dense and is an indicator of health. If there is no top edge or it is dark, the bone is not dense. This could indicate trouble.

Antibodies are protein molecules, which B-lymphocytes free so they can protrude from the exterior of pathogens, so they can be recognized and eliminated by other cells of the immune system.

Antigens activate the formation of antibodies and attach to the antibodies.

Calculus (tartar) is a hardened, porous buildup of mineral salts and dead bacteria. It mainly accumulates on the inside of the lower front teeth and the outside of the upper molars, near the saliva ducts. It may be many different colors: yellow, brown, black, orange or green, depending on how it developed. Calculus forms in places that routine brushing and flossing does not reach, making calculus a haven for bacteria.

Cementum is the thin layer that covers the roots of a tooth and contains fibers that are used as the attachment points for the periodontal ligament. Efforts should be made to avoid scraping this layer off of the roots. The cementum seals the dentinal tubes preventing bacteria from entering the root.

Cytotoxic T cells attack and literally blow up the infected cells by identifying antigens on the exterior of the cell.

Dentin is the layer below the enamel, which forms the body structure of the whole tooth. The dentin is composed of thousands of small tubes coursing out from the pulp surrounded by a bone like matrix. The tubes end at the enamel layer in the crown and the cementum layer in the root. There are approximately three miles of these tubes in each root. There is a normal flow of nutrients and fluid moving through these tubes from the inside to the outside of the tooth. These tubes are large enough to permit about seven bacteria to span a tube. If the outer protective layers are compromised it is possible for bacteria to enter the tubes.

Enamel of the crown is an approximately 98% crystalline layer of hydroxy apatite, a very hard form of calcium and other mineral salts. The concentration of trace minerals and the organic stains that seep between the mineral crystals determine the color of enamel.

Enamel is much harder than any other part of the tooth, creating a good surface to cut and grind food. Enamel is the hardest part of the human body; even harder than bone. The density of the enamel stops the most x-rays making it show up as the whitest part of the tooth. The cells that form enamel are lost when the tooth erupts into the mouth, so enamel cannot regenerate.

The major enemy of the enamel is acid. Enamel dissolves in a pH below 5.5 (water is approximately 7, cola is 2.5 and beer 4.5).

Gingivitis comes from "gingival" meaning gums and "itis" meaning inflammation. Gingivitis is an inflammation of the gums, usually accompanied by redness, swelling and easy bleeding. There is generally little or no discomfort at this stage. Gingivitis is usually reversible with professional treatment coupled with an effective oral hygiene and maintenance program at home. There is no bone or tooth loss. Pockets are under 3-4 mm. (3 mm equals 1/8 inch.)

Gum line is the scalloped, healthy level where the gums normally reach on teeth.

Infection is the invasion of body tissue by disease causing organisms.

Inflammatory reaction is a swelling and reddening of tissue that is a result of destructive enzymes and chemical messengers.

Lamina dura is the dense bony layer that directly attaches to the periodontal ligament and appears white on an x-ray. It should be visible on x-ray as a thin white line following and just outside of the dark line formed by the periodontal ligament. Often in a situation when there is an infection in the pulp of the tooth, the loss of the laminadura at the tip of the root is the first sign of trouble that can be seen on an x-ray.

Lymphocytes are a class of white blood cells, which boost immune function.

Macrophages are white blood cells that destroy pathogens by surrounding the pathogens and digesting them. Macrophages also display bits of the pathogens to other members of the defense system so they can identify them for destruction.

Periodontal ligament is the suspensor system that holds the tooth in the mouth. Contrary to common belief, teeth are not attached directly to the jawbones. Teeth rely on the ligament's fibers to cushion forces both in chewing and trauma. One end of the ligament attaches on the tooth root at the cementum. The other end of the ligament attaches to a dense layer of bone in the tooth socket called the lamina dura.

On an x-ray the periodontal ligament shows up as a thin dark line in healthy tissue. As the tooth loosens the periodontal ligament stretches and becomes wider. On an x-ray this stressed ligament shows up as a wider dark line. This indicates that the tooth has too much biting trauma.

Periodontitis is a combination of three Greek words: "peri" meaning around, "odont" referring to a tooth and "itis" which is inflammation. Periodontitis is inflammation around the tooth.

Plaque is a sticky water-repellent coating or bio-film on the teeth and gums. It is composed of food debris and over 500 forms of bacteria and their waste products. Plaque left on your teeth over 24 hours forms a matrix that attracts dissolved minerals in the saliva. This precipitation of mineral salts is the beginning of calculus. That is why it is very important to thoroughly brush your teeth at least once a day.

Pulp (the nerve) is the innermost layer of the tooth and consists of three important elements. First there are small arteries and veins to provide an adequate blood supply. Second, there is a nerve with primarily pain receptors. The only reaction that teeth have to any stimulus is pain. Third, there is a layer of cells that makes more of the dentin tooth structure as needed throughout life. The pulp appears dark on x-ray because the tissue is soft and not dense. Each root of a tooth has its own blood supply and nerve, and they all connect in the pulp chamber deep in the crown. These channels are called root canals.

T-Cells are a class of white blood cells that have many immune functions. They can destroy infected cells as well as stimulate the production of antibody from other cells. Their names comes from the thymus, where the cells are produced.

Tooth is a hard durable organ whose function is to chew all types of food. This represents the first step in the digestive process. There are 4 basic types of human teeth: incisors, cuspids, bicuspids and molars. They have special shapes and sizes adapting them to different chewing requirements.

The normally visible part of the tooth is the crown. The outer layer of the crown is the enamel. The high points are called cusps and the low valleys are called grooves. Below the enamel lies the dentin. Beneath the dentin is the inner-most layer, the pulp chamber. Hidden from sight, below the gums is the root. Like the crown, the root is composed of three layers, the outer layer called the cementum; the middle layer, a continuation of the dentin and the inner layer an extension of the pulp called the root canal.

White blood cells travel throughout the body's blood and lymph, directly or indirectly wiping out pathogens and infected cells.

Appendix B - Ingredients

Vitamin A is required for collegen synthesis. Vitamin A stimulates immunity and is needed for the formation of bone and wound healing.

Safety: Ingesting Vitamin A in excess of 50,000 IU may be toxic.[192]

Acetyl L-Carnitine works synergistically with CoQ10 and Alpha Lipoic Acid . It enhances cellular energy production in the mitochondria where ATP is made. Think of CoQ10 as the energy source, the mitochondria as the furnace and Acetyl L-Carnitine as the transportation device, delivering CoQ10 to the furnace.[193]

Aloe Vera acts as an astringent, emollient, antifungal, antibacterial and antiviral. Stimulates cell regeneration and reduces inflammation.[194]

Safety: Generally regarded as safe.

Alpha Lipoic Acid is a very potent antioxidant, sometimes referred as the universal antioxidant because it is soluble in both fat and water. It is also capable or regenerating other antioxidants, particularly CoQ10.[195]

Safety: Alpha Lipoic Acid is generally regarded as safe. Individuals with severe B12 deficiencies should avoid Alpha Lipoic Acid.

B Vitamins

Folic acid is an important PI fighting B vitamin. This is true for all individuals, especially for pregnant women and women on oral contraceptives who have high estrogen levels, which can create a folic acid deficiency.[250,251]

Mouthwashes with folic acid added may help offset folic acid deficiency more effectively than oral supplementation.[198,199,200,201]

Folic Acid is critical to cell division and new cell production because it is an essential co-factor in normal DNA synthesis. A deficiency of folic acid results in gum cells (epithelial cells) that do not divide properly, consequently a deficiency may predispose the tissue to PI. Also folic acid is a powerful free radical scavenger.[202,203]

Safety: Folic acid supplementation should always include B12 because folic acid can mask a B12 deficiency.

Vitamin B12 is added to formulas to insure that sufficient quantities are available.

Safety: Vitamin B12 has no known toxicity.

Vitamin B6, Folic Acid and Vitamin B12 are all important co-factors in the conversion of the amino acid methionine into cysteine. If these B vitamins are deficient, homocysteine increases. As homocysteine increases in the body it interferes with collagen cross-linking, leading to a defective bone matrix unable to hold calcium in the bone. Therefore all three of these B vitamins are critical to the building of healthy bones and teeth.[204,205,206,207]

Safety: Only B6 is associated with toxicity at doses greater than 2,000 mg, however an intake of more than 500 mg per day for several months can also become toxic. Folic acid should always include B12 because folic acid can mask a B12 deficiency.

Betaine Hydrochloric Acid (HCL) is essential for the conversion of methionine to cysteine. Deficiencies are associated with a negative effect on the collagen matrix of the bone.[208]

Safety: Betaine HCL is tolerated in the range of 100 to 500 mg per dose. Higher doses can cause acid irritation to the stomach lining.

Bio-Saponin is a proprietary extract of naturally occurring plant saponins. This substance is characterized by an ability to form emulsions and to foam in aqueous solutions. Bio-Saponin replaces the less costly and highly irritating foaming agent, sodium lauryl sulphate.

Safety: Generally regarded as safe.

Black Pepper Fruit (Piper Nigrum) is antimicrobial and significantly enhances the bioavailability of other nutrients through increased absorption.[209,210]

Safety: Black pepper Fruit is generally regarded as safe and nontoxic. The recommended amount of 5 mg per day is seven times less than the daily amount consumed by the average US citizen.[211]

Black Walnut Green Hull Extract is very effective at killing parasites. Specifically it is the green hull of the black walnut with critical attention to harvesting the hulls while green.[212]

Safety: Generally regarded as safe.

Blood Root Extract contains a primary alkaloid, sanguinarine, which is valuable in preventing the build-up of plaque. In vitro studies suggest that the plaque prevention occurs because sanguinarine keeps the bacteria from adhering to the teeth. Blood Root is also antimicrobial and anti-inflammatory.[213]

Safety: Generally regarded as safe.

Boron is an essential trace mineral in the prevention and treatment of bone loss. Research points out that boron alters the metabolism of other minerals. Boron also prevents excessive urinary excretion of calcium and magnesium.[214]

Safety: Boron is extremely safe when administered in the dosage range of 1 to 3 mg per day.

Vitamin C is the first line of antioxidant protection in the body and a powerful immune stimulant. In addition, it works synergistically with other substances by regenerating their oxidized states, because Vitamin C freely gives up its electrons.[215]

Vitamin C has a strong anti-histamine function thus reducing swelling, redness and pain, by directly detoxifying histamine or effecting a change in the level of enzymes responsible for histamine metabolism. Vitamin C is a co-factor in the collagen synthesis.[216]

Vitamin C also influences the longevity and activity level of a WBC's ability to destroy and digest toxins, bacteria and foreign matter within the tissue. Although some mammals can produce Vitamin C, humans must replenish their reserves on a regular basis. Many factors including stress and infection create a high demand for Vitamin C.[217,218]

Safety: Vitamin C is generally regarded as safe and non-toxic. Doses in excess of 1,000 mg can cause gas or diarrhea.[219] However, many people tolerate and benefit from much higher doses.

Calcium and magnesium in the proper ratio are very important for bone formation. Too much calcium inhibits magnesium, which is necessary for the production of the hormone calcitonin. Magnesium is essential for the conversion of vitamin D that is required for calcium absorption.[220,221]

Safety: Calcium and magnesium are generally well tolerated. However, calcium dosages should not exceed 2000 mg per day as higher dosages may increase the risk of kidney stones and soft-tissue deposition. Magnesium chloride, magnesium hydroxide or magnesium citrate are sometimes associated with loose stools.

Not all calcium supplements are alike. Certainly strong bones are needed in the mouth but not at the expense of substantially increased lead levels. Studies have indicated that calcium obtained from bone meal or oyster shell may contain considerable levels of lead.[222]

Calendula (marigold) is astringent and is soothing to the skin. It is an anti-fungal and reduces inflammation.[223]
Safety: Calendula is considered safe for external use.

Cinnamon Oil controls the growth of C. albicans, E. coli and Staph aureus. Chemical studies show that a component of cinnamon, cinnamaldehyde react with bacteria shifting the growth of bacterial cells to an unbalanced state, thus inhibiting cell viability. This highly anti-microbial essential oil has been used in Sri Lanka for over 2,000 years.[224,225,226]
Safety: Generally regarded as safe.

Clove Oil is highly antimicrobial, antiseptic, analgesic, bactericidal, antioxidant and anti-inflammatory.[227,228,229,230]
Safety: Generally regarded as safe.

CoEnzyme Q10 (CoQ10) is extremely important in the repair and maintenance of periodontal tissue. It is the energy carrier of ATP. Several studies point out the correlation between PI and CoQ10 deficiencies. CoQ10 is a powerful antioxidant and without enough CoQ10 to boost resistance, a person's periodontal damage may exceed repair.[231,232,233,234]

Applying CoQ10 directly to the gums coupled with adequate supplementation can reverse most conditions.[235,236,237]

Unlike many prescription and alternative solutions to health problems, the results of CoQ10 are quickly observed.[238]

Safety: CoEnzymeQ10 is generally regarded as safe and non-toxic. Because safety during pregnancy and lactation has not been proven CoQ10 is not recommended unless the medical outcome of attacking PI outweighs the risk of using CoQ10.

Copper like zinc is an essential constituent of many important body enzymes including a form of super oxide dismutase (SOD), a major cellular antioxidant that cannot be supplemented directly. Copper is required by the body to produce hemoglobin, the oxygen carrier in our blood.[239]

Safety: Most people receive sufficient amounts of copper in their diet, and too much copper can product free radicals. However, individuals consuming high levels of fructose and high levels of zinc should balance it with small levels of copper.

Vitamin D is essential for calcium metabolism and required for strong teeth formation. Vitamin D has hormone-like properties that directs serum calcium to the bone and suppress excess parathyroid hormone levels that can pull calcium from the bone.[240]

Safety: Prolonged consumption of Vitamin D in excess of 1000 iu per day maybe toxic.

Vitamin E has powerful wound healing properties and can improve circulation in the tiniest capillaries. It is equally important as an antioxidant, as it prevents oxidation of lipids (fats).[241,242,243]

Echinacea's protective action inhibits the breakdown of hyaluronic acid (a glue-like substance that holds the matrix of connective tissue together). Hyaluronic acid functions as a barrier preventing bacteria from spreading. Echinacea can also stimulate certain cells (fibroblasts) to produce new connective tissue.[244,245,246]

This herb possesses direct anti-inflammatory effects. The entire immune system is stimulated by Echinacea's ability to increase the number and the lifespan of WBCs in the area that requires healing. Echinacea also has a direct enhancing effect on the secretion of adrenal cortisone.[247,248,249]

The Echinacin B fraction isolate is important because of its antihyaluronidase activity promotes wound healing and cell renewal.[250]

Safety: Echinacea is generally regarded as safe and non-toxic.

Eucalyptus Oil is a powerful anti-microbial agent. Eucalyptus globules, which contains a high percentage of eucalyptus oil, is very antiseptic. This is the reason why eucalyptus is found in many mouth rinses. It is also anti-fungal. For hundreds of years, Australian Aborigines used eucalyptus leaves as a disinfectant to cover wounds.[251]

Safety: Generally regarded as safe.

Gota Kola (centella asiatica) increases blood supply to connective tissue. It promotes rapid wound healing by accelerating tissue growth. It also exhibits an antimicrobial action by dissolving the waxing covering of certain viruses and bacteria.[252,253,254,255,256]

Safety: Generally regarded as safe.

Grapefruit Seed Extract has been proven to be antibacterial, anti-viral and anti-fungal by the University of Georgia at Athens.[257]

Safety: Generally regarded as safe.

Grape seed (*vitis vinifera*) is a source of OPCs (oligomeric proanthocyanidins complexes), which plays a major role in preventing PI by coating the bacterial membranes so they cannot group together. This process keeps the bacteria from forming plaque.[258]

OPCs also have many mechanisms that help control PI. They protect the collagen and elastin of our connective tissue from the free radicals produced by bacteria and white blood cells.[259,260] They also inhibit destructive enzymes such as collagenase and serine protease, which when released by white blood cell (WBCs) and bacteria, dissolve collagen. They also inhibit hyaluronidase, which allows the spread of infection by breaking down hyaluronic acid (the glue-like substance that holds the matrix of connective tissue together).[261,262,263,264]

Histamine can help the body by protecting against the excessive release of harmful enzymes. Unfortunately histamine has the adverse effect of causing swelling, redness and pain. Grape seed extract blocks this excessive production of histamine.[265,267] OPCs are also free radical scavengers, twenty times greater than vitamin C and fifty times greater than vitamin E.[268]

Safety: Grape seed extract has no toxic side effects with the exception of temporary skin irritation of people who are sensitive to grapes.[269]

Vitamin K is a hormone-like vitamin needed to retain calcium within the bone matrix and also helps blood to clot. In both situations its role is to transport calcium to where it is needed in the body. It has been called the "anti-hemorrhagic" vitamin.[270]

Safety: Vitamin K may interfere with some prescription blood thinners. Vitamin K is not stored in the liver.

Lavender Oil is antiseptic, antimicrobial and anti-inflammatory.[271,272,273,274,275]

Safety: Generally regarded as safe.

Lysine is an essential amino acid that form about 12% of the collagen and elastin in the human body. When lysine is supplied in sufficient amounts as a dietary supplement, it can block the anchor sites in the connective tissue that collagenase, a collagen-destroying enzyme, uses to attach to the tissue. In this way lysine prevents this enzyme from uncontrollably disintegrating connective tissue. Lysine is also the basic building block of the amino acid carnitine.[276]

Safety: Even increased dosages of lysine are considered safe because our bodies are accustomed to large amounts. Lysine usage should be accompanied with proline and B6.

Manganese has been shown to specifically act as a catalyst in the development and maintenance of the organic bone matrix. A deficiency of manganese may lead to tooth grinding.[281]

Safety: Manganese is generally regarded as safe and nontoxic in small doses.

Molybdenum is involved in the biochemical processes of cellular respiration and utilization of oxygen, maintenance of cell membrane integrity and capturing free radicals. This mineral is important in supporting the enzyme process of converting toxic sulfides, a common preservative, to safer sulfates, which can then be excreted in the urine. An Austrian study of 1,750 patients found that 41.5 percent were molybdenum-deficient.[282]

Safety: Molybdenum is generally regarded as safe and nontoxic in small doses. Extremely high doses may lead to the development of gout.

Methionine is an essential amino acids (building blocks of protein). It supplies sulfur required for normal metabolism and growth. By inactivating free radicals, methionine becomes a powerful antioxidant.[283]

Safety: Methionine is generally regarded as safe as long as adequate amounts of B Vitamins are taken.

Olive Leaf (oleuropein) **Oleopein**® is a powerful antibacterial, antiviral and antiparasitic. The main active ingredient is a substance called elenolic acid, which inactivates bacteria by dissolving their outer cell wall. It neutralizes viral replication by interfering with critical amino acid replications essential to the viruses. It has also been found effective in controlling fungal, yeast and mold infections.[284,285,286]

Through extensive testing, it was discovered that olive leaf extract has other unique properties. It contains components called iridoids that create a structurally complicated molecule, which bugs cannot readily develop a resistance to. Another important fact is that it does not destroy the beneficial bacteria in the intestines.[287,288]

Safety: Olive leaf extract has been found to be safe in amounts far higher than the normal daily amount. Scientific testing indicates that amounts many times larger than the daily recommended safe doses are not toxic and do not cause adverse side effects.

Oregano Oil in many studies is credited with total inhibition of microorganisms, including *Staphylococcus aureus, Escherichia coli (E coli), Pseudomonas aeruglinosa* and *Aspergillus niger.* This powerful immune stimulant herb has a broad range of antimicrobial activities against fungus, virus and bacteria.[289,290,291,292,293,294,295,296]

Safety: Generally regarded as safe.

Peppermint Oil is an anti-carcinogenic, anti-parasite and anti-inflammatory.[297,298,299]

Safety: Generally regarded as safe.

Phytoplenolin® is a holistically balanced and patented Bio-Botanica® preparation of the herb, Centiepeda cunninghami. It has been demonstrated in laboratory and clinical studies to be both a powerful anti-viral and anti-inflammatory. As well, this relative of the daisy family is an effective cell renewal (healing) agent. Other effects cited in the literature are antihistaminic and antimutigenic. Properties attributed to Phytophenolin® are substantiated in extensive research studies conducted by outside testing laboratories.[300,301,302,303]

Plant enzymes improve the bioavailability of other supplements.[304]
Safety: Plant enzymes are generally regarded as safe and nontoxic.

Prickly Ash Bark increases capillary circulation.[305]
Safety: Generally regarded as safe.

Proline is a non-essential amino acid, which the body can make on its own. However since lysine and proline make-up such a large percentage of collagen, it is important to provide adequate amounts when taking increased quantities of lysine.[306]

Quercetin is a bioflavonoid. It is a powerful anti-inflammatory that is known to inhibit mast cells (histamine producing cells) from releasing inflammatory compounds.[307,308,309]
Safety: Quercetin is generally regarded as safe.

Rhatany is an astringent herb, which may help to stop bleeding.[310]
Safety: Generally regarded as safe.

Selenium plays a vital role in the functioning of the antioxidant enzyme glutathione peroxidase. As such, it affects all components of the immune system, including the development and activity of all WBCs.
A deficiency has been shown to inhibit resistance to infection as a result of impaired WBC and thymus function, while

selenium supplementation has been shown to stimulate WBC and thymus function. Apparently, selenium supports the expression of the immune-enhancing compound Interleukin-II and, consequently the rate of WBC proliferation and differentiation into forms capable of killing microorganisms.[311,312]

Safety: Selenium is generally regarded as safe and nontoxic in very small doses.

Silica is the most commonly found form of the element silicon. Silica plays an essential role in the cross linking mechanism in collagen formation, the connective tissue matrix of bone. Recalcification in bone remodeling may be dependent on adequate levels of silica. The best-documented function of silica is the acceleration of bone regeneration by aiding in the deposit of calcium and other minerals.[313,314]

Safety: Silica is generally regarded as safe and nontoxic.

Thyme Oil has been used for centuries for infections of all kinds. It is anti-microbial, with positive actions against bacteria, viruses and fungus.[315,316,317,318,319,320,321,322]

Safety: Generally regarded as safe.

Xylitol is a remarkable substance. It is all natural, produced by the human body in small amounts, is FDA rated safe for babies without restriction. It fights cavities, plaque, dry mouth, bad breath, and neutralizes bacterial acids, and even remineralizes tooth enamel. Xylitol works by washing away bacteria not killing them like antibiotics do.[323]

Safety: Generally regarded as safe.

Zinc methionate is the most bioavailable form of zinc. This mineral's importance in treating PI cannot be overstated. Zinc functions synergistically with Vitamin A in many body processes. Decreased zinc levels directly correlate with the severity of PI. It is essential for the formation of superoxide dismutase (SOD), one of body's most important free radical scavengers. SOD cannot be directly supplemented because it is poorly absorbed. Zinc also promotes wound healing, immune function, taste sensitivity, protein synthesis and insulin production.[324,325]

Safety: Generally regarded as safe and nontoxic in small doses.

Literature Cited

1. Page, R.C., and H. Schroeder. 1982. *Periodontitis in man and other animals, a comparative review.* Basal: S. Karger.

2. Page, R.C. 1991. *The role of inflammatory mediators in the pathogensis of periodontal disease. J. Periodont Res.* 26:230-42.

3. Williams, R. 1998. Periodontal disease: the emergence of a new paradigm. *Compend Contin Educ Dent Supp.* 19:4-10.

4. Rose, L.R., B.J. Steinberg and L. Minsk. 2000. The relationship between periodontal disease and systemic conditions. *Compendium* 10: 870-877.

5. Meinig, G.E. 1998. *Root Canal Cover-up.* Ojai, Calif.: Bion Publishing.

6. Glassman, G. 1998. Root canal cover-up exposed: the resurgence of the refuted focal infection theory. *Oral Health* 88 (12): 3.

7. Debelian, et al. 1998. Anaerobic bacteremia and fungemia in patients undergoing endodontic therapy: an overview. *Ann Periodontogy* 3 (1): 281-7.

8. *Oral Health in America. A report of the Surgeon General. Executive Summary.* Department of Health and Human Services.

9. Golub. 1998. *Dentistry Today* (Oct).

10. Navazesh, M and R Mulligan. 1995. Systemic dissemination as a result of oral infection in individuals 50 years of age and older. *Spec. Care Dentist* 15 (1): 11-9.

11. Page, R.C. and K.S. Kornman. 1997. The pathogenesis of human periodontitis: an introduction. *Periodontol 2000* 14:.9-11.

12. Loe, et al. 1986. Natural history of periodontal disease in man: rapid, moderate and no loss of attachment in Sri Lankan laborers 14 to 46 years of age. *J. Clin. Periodontol* 13:431-445.

13. Chen, I. 2000. The Surgeon General's report on oral health: implications for research and education. *NY State Den.t J.* 66:.38-42.

14. Lamont, R.J. and H.F. Jenkinson. 1998. Life below the gum line: pathogenic mechanism of *Porphyromonas Gingivalis. Microbiol. Mo.l Biol. Rev.* 62 (4):.1244-63.

15. Debekuan, et al. 1994. Systemic diseases caused by oral microorganisms. *Endod. Dent. Traumato.* 10 (2): 57-65.

16. Beck, et al. 1998. Periodontitis: a risk factor for coronary heart disease. *Ann. Periodontol.* 3 (1): 127-41.

17. Loesche, W. 1997. Associations of the oral flora with important medical diseases. *Current Opinion Periodontal* 4:21-8.

18. Meyer, D.H. and P.M. Fives-Taylor. 1998. Oral pathogens: from dental plaque to cardiac disease. *Current Opinion Microbiol.* 1 (1):88-95.

19. Dorn, et al. 1999. Invasion of human coronary artery cells by periodontal pathogens. *Infection and Immunity* 67 (11): 5792-5798.

20. Emingil, G et al. 2000. Association between periodontal disease and acute myocardial infarction. *Journal of Periodontology* 71 (12): 1882-1886.

21. Iacopino, et al. 2000. Pathophysiological relationships between Periodontitis and systemic disease: Recent concepts involving serum lipids. *Journal of Periodontology* 71 (8): 1375-1384.

22. Haraszthy, et al. 1999. Identification of periodontal pathogens in atheromatous plaques. *J. Periodontol 2000* 71(10): 1554-60.

23. Wu, T. 2000. Periodontal disease and risk of cerebrovascular disease: the first national health and nutrition examination survey and its follow-up study. *American Journal of Epidemiology* 151: 273-282.

24. DeNardin, et al. 2000. Fibrinogen linked to gum disease. U. of Buffalo 31 (27).

25. Genco, R.J. 1999. *Risk factors for periodontal diseases. Periodontal Medicine.* Ontario, Canada: BC Decker Publishing.

26. Loesch, W.J. 1994. Periodontal disease as a risk factor for heart desease. *Compendium* 15(8): 976,978-82,985-6 passim; quiz 992.

27. Joshipura, K.J. 1996. Poor oral health and coronary heart disease. *J. Dent. Res.* 75 (9): 1631-6.

28. Syrjanen, et al. 1989. Dental infections in association with cerebral infarction in young and middle-age men. *J. Intern. Med.* 225(3): 179-84.

29. Beck, et al. 1996. Periodontal disease and cardiovascular disease. *J. Periodontol.* 67 (suppl.1): 1123-37.

30. Ibid.

31. Arbes, et al. 1999. Association between extent of periodontal attachment loss and self-reported history of heart attack: an analysis of NHANES III date *J. Dent. Res.* 798 (12): 1777-82.

32. Herzberg, M.C. and M.W. Meyer. 1996. Effects of oral flora on platelets: possible consequences in cardiovascular disease. *J. Periodontol* 67 (10 Suppl): 1138-42.

33. Herzberg, M.C. and M.W. Meyer. 1998. Dental plaque, platelets and cardiovascular diseases. *Ann. Periodontol* 3 (1): 151-60.

34. Dorn, B.R. et al. 1999. Invasion of human coronary artery cells by periodontal pathogens. *Infect. Immun.* 67 (11): 5792-5798.

35. Mattila, et al. 1993. Dental Infections as a risk factor for acute myocardial infarction. *Eur. Heart J.* 14 (Suppl K): 51-3.

36. Mattila, et al. 1993. Dental infections and coronary atherosclerosis. *Atherosclerosis* 103 (2):205-11.

37. Mattila, et al. 1995. Dental infection and the risk of new coronary events: prospective study of patients with documented coronary artery disease. *Clin. Infect. Dis.* 20 (3):588-92.

38. Wu, et al. 2000. Periodontal disease and risk of cerebrovascular disease: the First National Health and Nutrition Examination Survey and its follow-up study. *Archives of Internal Medicine* 18:2749-2755.

39. Grau, et al. 1997. Association between acute cerebrovascular ischemia and chronic and recurrent infection. *Journal Stroke* (9) 1724-9.

40. Grossi, et al. 1997. Treatment of periodontal disease in diabetics reduces glycated hemoglobin. *J. Periodontol* 68(8): 713-719.

41. Grossi, et al. 1998. Periodontal Disease and Diabetes Mellitius: A two-way relationship. *Annals Periodontol* 3(1): 51-61.

42. Thorstensson, et al. 1996. Medical status and complications in relation to periodontal disease experience in insulin-dependent diabetics. *J. Clin. Periodontol* 23 (3 Pt 1): 194-202.

43. Shlossman, et al. 1990. Type 2 diabetes mellitus and periodontal disease. *J. Am. Dent. Assoc.* 121:532-536.

44. Murayama, et al. 2001. The effect of antimicrobial periodontal treatment on circulating tumor necrosis factor-alpha and glycated hemoglobin level in patients with type 2 diabetes. *Journal of Periodontol* 72 (6): 774-778.

45. Katz, J. 2001. Elevated blood glucose levels in patients with severe periodontal disease. *J. Clin. Periodontol* 28: 710-12.

46. Nelson, et al. 1990. Periodontal disease and NIDDM in Pima Indians. *Diabetes Care* 13:836-40.

47. Tabaj, et al. 2000. Flow cytometry as a new method to study periodontal disease in diabetic patients. *Diabetologia Croatica.* 29 (1): 27-31.

48. *National Diabetes Data Group: Diabetes in America data compiled 1984.* 1985. Bethesda, Md. National Institute of Health. Publication No. 851268.

49. Heller, et al. *The Carbohydrate Addict's Healthy Heart Program.* New York: Ballantine Books.

50. Ibid.

51. Grossi, et al. 2000. Obesity-gum disease link found. *U of Buffalo Reporter* 31 (25).

52. Ibid.

53. O'Abay. 1996. Does H. pylori induce gastritis food-stimulated insulin release? *Dig. Dis. Sci.* 41 (7): 21327-31.

54. Scannapieco, F.A., and J.M. Mylotte. 1996. Relationships between periodontal disease and bacterial pneumonia. *J. Periodontol* 67(10 Suppl): 114-22.

55. Dahlen, et al. 1995. Occurrence of enteric rods, staphylococci and Candida in subgingival samples. *Oral Microbio.l Immunol.*10:42-46.

56. Bentley, D.W. 1984. Bacterial pneumonia in the elderly: clinical features, diagnosis, etiology and treatment. *Gerontol.* 30:297-307.

57. Dasanayake, A.P. 1998. Poor periodontal health of the pregnant woman as a risk factor for low birth weight. *Ann. Periodontol* 3 (1):206-12.

58. Davenport, et al. 1998. The East London study of maternal chronic periodontal disease and pre-term low birth weight infants: study design and prevalence data. *Ann Periodontol* 3 (1): 213-21.

59. Offenbacher, et al. 1998. Potential pathogenic mechanisms of periodontitis associated pregnancy complications. *Ann Periodontol* 3(1):233-50.

60. Offenbacher, et al. 1996. Periodontal disease as a possible risk factor for pre-term low birth weight. *J. Periodontal* 67:1103-13.

61. Gibbs, et al. 1992. A review of premature birth and subclinical infections. *American Journal Obster. Gynecol.* 166(5): 1515-1528.

62. Loesche, W.J. 1997. Association of the oral flora with important medical diseases. *Curr. Opin. Periodontol* 4:21-28.

63. American Academy of Periodontology Specialty Conference on Periodontal Medicine, Importance of Good Oral Health in Pregnant Women. 2000. Washington D.C.

64. Hill, G.B. 1998. Preterm birth: associations with genital and possibly oral microflora. *Ann. Periodontol.* 3(1): 222-32.

65. Collins, et al. 1994. Effects of *Porphyromonas Gingivalis* infection on inflammatory mediator response and pregnancy outcome in hamster. *Infect. Immun.* 62:4356-4361.

66. Collins, et al. 1994. Effects of *Escherichia coli* and *Porphyromonas gingivalis* lipopolysaccharide on pregnancy outcome in the golden hamster. *Infect. Immun.* 62:4652-4655.

67. Tezak, et al. 2000. The relationship between bone mineral density and periodontitis in postmenopausal women. *J Periodontol.* 71(9): 1492-1498.

68. Loomer, et al. 1994. Direct effects of metabolic products and sonicated extracts of *Porphyromonas Gingivalis* 2561 on ostergenesis in vitro. *Infect. Immune.* 62(4) :1289-97.

69. Wactawski-Wende, et al. 1998. Osteoporosis, oral health linked ; Analysis of national database shows strong relationship. *American Association for the Advancement of Science.*

70. Ebersole, J.L. 1990. Systemic humoral immune response in periodontal disease. *Crit. Rev. Oral. Biol. Med.* 1:283-331.

71. Moore, W.E.C., and L.V.H. Moore. 1994.The bacteria of periodontal diseases. *Periodontol 2000* 5:66-77.

72. Page, R.C. 1991.The role of inflammatory mediators in the pathogenesis of periodontal disease. *J. Periodont. Res.* 26:230-242.

73. Holt, S.C., and T.E. Bramanti. 1991. Factors in virulence expression and their role in periodontal disease pathogenesis. *Crit. Rev. Oral. Biol. Med.* 2:177-281.

74. Haffajee, A.D., and S.S. Socransky. 1994. Microbial etiologic agents of destructive periodontal diseases. *Periodontol 2000* 5:78-111.

75. Lamont, R.J., and H.F. Jenkinson. 1998. Life below the gum line: pathogenic mechanisms of *Porphyromonas gingivalis*. *Microbiol. Rev.* 62(4): 1244-63.

76. Wilson, M., and B. Henderson. 1995. Virulence factors of Actinobacillus actinomycetemcomitans relevant to the pathogenesis of inflammatory periodontal diseases. *FEMS Microbiol. Rev.* 17:365-379.

77. Fives-Taylor, P., D. Meyer, and K. Mintz. 1995. Characteristics of Actinobacillus actinomycetemcomitans invasion of and adhesion to cultured epithelial cells. *Adv. Dent. Res.* 9:55-62.

78. Lamont, et al. 1995. *P. gingivalis* invasion of gingival epithehal cells. *Infect. Immun.* 63:3878-3885.

79. Cugini, et al. 2000. The effect of scaling and root planning on the clinical and microbiological parameters of periodontal disease: 12-month results. *J. Clin. Periodontol.* 27(1): 30-6.

80. Haffajee, A.D., and S.S. Socransky. 1994. Microbial etiologic agents of destructive periodontal diseases. *Periodontol 2000* 5:78-111.

81. Lavine, et al. 1979. Impaired neutrophil chemotaxis in patients with juvenile and rapidly progressing periodontitis. *J. Periodont. Res.* 14:10-19.

82. Van Dyke, et al. 1983. Juvenile periodontitis as a model for neutrophil function: reduced binding of complement chemotactic fragment. *J. Den. Res.* 62:870-872.

83. Concensus report on Periodontal diseases: pathogenesis and microbial factors. 1996. *Ann Periodontol* 1: 926-932.

84. Gillespie, et al. Isolation and partial characterization of the *Campylobacter rectus* cytotoxin.

85.Schenkein, H.A. 1989. Failure of Bacteroides Gingivalis W83 to accumulate bound C3 following opsonization with serum. *J. Periodont. Res.* 24:20-27.

86. Culter, C.N., R.R. Arnold and H.A. Schenkein 1993. Inhibition of C3 and IgG proteolysis enhances phagocytosis of *Porphyromonas gingivalis*. *J. Immunol.* 151:7016-7029.

87. Shenker, B.J., L.A.Vitale and D.A. Welham. 1990. Immune suppression induced by *Actinobacillus actinomycetemcomitans*: Effects on immunoglobulin prodiction by human B cells. *Infect. Immun.* 58:3856-3862.

88. Offenbacher, S. 1996. Periodontal diseases: Pathogenesis. *Ann. Periodontol.* 1:821-878.

89. Reynolds, J.J., and M.C. Meikle. 1997. Mechanism of connective tissue destruction in periodontitis. *Periodontol 2000.* 14:144-157.

90. Birkedal-Hansen, H. 1993. Role of cytokines and inflammatory mediators in tissue destruction. *J. Periodont Res.* 28:500-510.

91. Goldhaber, et al. 1973. Bone reabsorption in tissue culture and its relevance to periodontal disease. *J. Am. Dent. Assoc.* 87:1027-1033.

92. Moore, W.E.C., and L.V.H. Moore. 1994. The bacteria of periodontal diseases. *Periodontol 2000.* 5:66-77.

93. Miyasaki, K.T. 1001. The neutrophil: Mechanisms of controlling periodontal bacteria. *J. Periodontol.* 2:761-774.

94. Ebersole, J.L. 1990. Systemic humoral immune responses in periodontal disease. *Crit. Rev. Oral. Biol. Med.*1:283-331.

95. Llamster, I.B. and M.J. Novak. 1992. Host mediators in gingival crevicular fluid: Implications for the pathogenesis of periodontal disease. *Crit. Rev. Oral. Bio. Med.* 3:31-60.

96. Allison, et al. 1976. Activation of complement by the alternative pathway as a factor in the pathogenesis of periodontal disease. *Lancet* 2 (7993):1001-4.

97. Schindler, L.W. How the Immune System works. *National Institute of Health.*

98. Genco, et al. 2000. Low Dietary Vitamin C Can Increase Risk for Periodontal disease. *J. of Periodontology.*

99. Grossi et al. 1999. HNANES III. *University of Buffalo Reporter.* 30 (24).

100. Mcguire, M.K., and M.M. Nunn. 1999. The effectiveness of clinical parameters and IL-1 genotype in accurately predicting prognoses and tooth survival. *J. Periodontol* 70 (1): 49-56.

101. Komman, et al. 1997. The interleukin-1 genotype as a severity factor in adult periodontal disease. *J. Clin. Periodontol* 24:72-77.

102. Hart, T., and K.S. 1997. Komman. Genetic factors in the pathogensis of periodontitis. *Periodontol 2000* 14:202-215.

103. World Health Organization: The World Health Report 1995: bridging the gap. Geneva, Switzerland.

104. Gallin, J.L. 1988. *The neutrophil: Immunological diseases.* 4th ed. Boston: Little, Brown.

105. Pisciotta, A.V. 1990. Drug-induced agranulocytosis; peripheral destruction of polymorphonuclear leukocytes and their marrow precursors. *Blood Rev.* 4(4): 226-37.

106. Nery, et al. 1995. Prevalence of nifedipine-induced gingival hyperplasis. *J. Periodontol.* 66:572-578.

107. Tomar, S.L. and S. Asma. 2000. Smoking - attributable periodontitis in the United States findings for NHANES III. *J. Periodontol 2000.* 71:743-751.

108. Gelsky, S.C. 1999. Cigarette smoking and periodontitis: Methodology to assess the strength of evidence in support of a causal association. *Comm. Dent. Oral. Epidemiol.* 27:16-24.

109. Costerton, et al. 1994. Biofilms, the customized microniche. *J. Bacteriol.* 176:2137-2142.

110. Haber, J. 1994. Cigarette smoking: a major risk factor for periodontitis. *Compend. Contin. Dent. Educ.* 15:1002-14.

111. Edwardsson, et al. 1999. The microbiota of periodontal pockets with different depths in the therapy-resistant periodontitis. *J. Clin. Periodontol.* 26(3): 143-52.

112. Tomar, S.L., and S. Asma. 2000. Smoking-attributable periodontitis in the United States: findings for NHANES III. *J. Periodontol 2000* 71:743-751.

113. Ibid.

114. Grossi, et al. 2001. Caution: alcohol may be hazardous to your (oral) health. *UB Research Quarterly* (Feb).

115. Watson, M.R., W.A. Bretz, and W. J. Loesche. 1994. Presence of *Treponema denticola* and *Porphyromonas gingivalis* in children correlated with periodontal disease of their parents. *Journal of Dental Research.* 73(10): 1636-40.

116. Petit, et al. 1994. Prevalance of periodontitis and suspected periodontal pathogens in families of adult periodontitis paients. *J. Clin. Periodontol.* 21: 76-85.

117. van Steenbergen, et al. 1993. Transmission of *Porphyromonas gingivalis* between spouses. *J. Clin Periodontol* 20:340-5.

118. Preus, et al. 1994. The distribution and transmission of *Actinobacillus actinomycetemcomitans* in families with established adult periodontitis. *Journal Periodontol.* 65:2-7.

119. Saarela, et al. 1993. Transmission of oral bacterial species between spouses. *Oral. Microbiol. Immunol.* 8:349-54.

120. Asikainen, S., C. Chen and J. Slots. 1996. Likelihood of transmitting *Actinobacillus actinomycetemcomitans* and *Porphyromonas gingivalis* in families with periodontitis. *Oral Microbiol Immunol.* 11(6): 387-94.

121. Asikainen, S. and C. Chen. 1999. Oral ecology and person-to-person transmission of *Actinobacillus actinomycetemcomitans* and *Porphyromonas gingivalis. Periodontol 2000.* 20:65-81.

122. Preus, H.R. and L. Olsen. 1988. Possible transmittance of *A. actinomycetemcomitans* from a dog to a child with rapidly destructive periodontitis. *Journal of Periodontal Research* 23:68-71.

123. Barker, K.F. 1999. Antibiotic resistance: a current perspective. *Br. J. Clin. Pharmacol.* 48:109-24.

124. Roberts, M.C. 1998. Antibiotic resistance in oral/respiratory bacteria. *Crit. Rev. Oral. Biol. Med.* 9(4): 522-40.

125 Summers, A. et al. 1993. Mercury released from Dental"silver" fillings provokes and increase in mercury-and antibiotic-resistant bacteria in oral and intestinal floras of primates. *Antimicrob. Agents Chemother.* 37(4): 825-34.

126. Lorsheider, et al. 1995. The dental amalgam mercury controversy-inorganic mercury and the CNS; genetic linkage of mercury and antibiotic resistances in intestinal bacteria. *Toxicology* 31(1-3):19-22.

127. Edlund, et al. 1996. Resistance of the normal human microflora to mercury and antimicrobials after exposure to mercury from dental amalgam fillings. *Clin. Infect. Dis.* 22(6): 944-50.

128. Smith, A., and J. Bragg. 1998. An update on antimicrobial chemotherapy 3: antimicrobial resistance and the oral cavity. *Dental Update.* 25:230-4.

129. van Windelhoff, A.J. et al. 2000. Antimicrobial resistance in the subfingival microflora in patients with adult periodontitis: a comparison between the Netherlands and Spain. *J Clin Periodontol* 27 (2)79-86.

130. Fives-Taylor, P.M. et al. 1999. Virulence factors of *Actinobacillus actinomycetemcomitans*. *Periodontol 2000* 20:136-67.

131. Larsen, T. 1991. Occurrence of doxycycline-resistant bacteria in the oral cavity after administration of doxycycline in patients with periodontal disease. *Scand J Infect Dis.* 23:89-96.

132. Ibid.

133. Rosenberg, J. 2000. Antibiotic resistance: what physicians should know. *Division of Communicable Disease Control: California Department of Health Services* January.

134. Ballow, C. 1998. Antibiotics vs. infectious bacteria: a battlefield report. *U. of Buffalo Reporter* 29 (21) February.

135. Williams, D. 2000. A new edge in the race against thoroughbred bugs. *Alternatives.* Vol.8. no.17 Nov.

136. Ballow, C. 1998. Antibiotics vs. infectious bacteria: a battlefield report. *U. of Buffalo Reporter* 29 (21) February.

137. Levy, S.B. 1992. *The Antibiotic Paradox: How Miracle Drugs Are Destroying the Miracle.* New York: Plenum Publishing.

138. Walker, CB. 1996. The acquisition of antibiotic resistance in periodontal microflora. *Periodontol 2000.* 10:79-88.

139. Baker, P. et al. 1995. Antibiotic susceptibility of anaerobic bacteria from the human cavity. *J Dent Res.* 64:1233-44.

140. Walker, C.B. et al. 1983. Antibody susceptibility testing of subgingival plaque samples. *J Clin Periodontol* 10:422-432.

141. Lewis, M.A. et al. 1995. Prevalence of penicillin resistant bacteria in acute suppurative oral infection. *J Antimicrob Chemother.* 35:785-91.

142. Sorsa, T. et al. 1992. Cellular source and tetracycline inhibition of gingival crevicular fluid collagenase of patients with labile diabetes mellitus. *J Clin Periodontol* 19 (2):146-149.

143. Grant, D, *Infectious Disease and Super Germs.*

144. Strom, B.L. et al. 1998. Dental and cardiac risk factors for infective endocarditis: a population-based-control study. *Ann Intern Med.* 129:761-9.

145. Durack, D.T. et al. 1983. Apparent failures of endocarditis prophylaxis. *JAMA* 250:2318-22.

146. American Academy of Periodontology. 1996. Systemic antibiotics in periodontics (position paper). *J Periodontol.* 67:831-8.

147. Ewald, P. 2000. *Plaque Time.* New York: The Free Press.

148. Wilson, T.G. Jr. 1996. Supportive periodontal treatment introduction: definition, extent of need, therapeutic objectives, frequency and efficacy. *Periodontol 2000* 12:11-15.

149. Lamster, I.B. 2001. Current Concepts and Future Trends for Periodontal Disease and Periodontal Therapy, Part 2. *Dentistry Today.* 3:88.

150. Estafen, et al. 1999. Adjunctive diagnostic methods for monitoring progressive periodontal diseases. *Gen Dent.* 47 (4):374-80.

151. Mancina, S. et al. 1999. Assessment of a novel screening test for Neutrophil collagenase activity in the diagnosis of periodontal diseases. *J Periodontol.* 70 (11):1292-302.

152. Slots, J. 1996. Microbial analysis in supportive periodontal therapy. *Periodontol 2000.* 12:56-9.

153. Loesche, W. et al. 1992. Comparison of the benzoyl-DL-arginine-naphthylamide (BANA) test, DNA probes, and immunologicalreagents for ability to detect anaerobic periodontal infections due to Porphyroomonas gingivalis,*Treponema denticola* and Bacteroides forsythus. *J Clin Microbiol.* 30:427-433.

154. Loesche, W. et al. 1997. The optimization of the BANA test as a screening agent for gingivitis among subjects seeking dental treatment. *J Clin Perio.* 4:114.

155. Lindhe, J. et al. 1982. Critical probing depths in periodontal therapy. *J Clin Periodontol.* 9(4): 323-36.

156. Riffle, A.B. 1952. The cementum during curettage. *J Periodontol.* 23:170-177.

157. BBC Homepage. 2001. *Health news.* Thursday, 26 July.

158. Dyer, D, Addy M, Newcombe R.G. 2000. Studies in vitro of abrasion by different manual toothbrush heads and a standard toothpaste. *J Clin Periodontol.* 27 (2) 99-103.

159. Warren, D. et al. 2001. The effects of toothpastes on the residual microbial contamination of toothbrushes. *Journal of the American Dental* 9:1241-1245.

160. Cobb, C.M. 1920. Toothbrushes as a cause of repeated infections of the mouth. *Boston Medical Surgery Journal* 183:263-4.

161. Glass, R.T. and S. Shapiro. 1993. Oral inflammatory disease and the toothbrush. *J Ala Dent Assoc.* 77(4): 12-6.

162. Glass, R.T. 1992. The infected toothbrush, the infected denture and transmission of disease: a review. *Compendium* 13(7): 592-8.

163. Svanberg, M. 1978. Contamination of toothpaste and toothbrush by *Streptococcus mutans. Scand J Dent Res* 86:412-4.

164. Kozai, K., T. Iwai and D. Miura. 1989. Residual contamination of toothbrushes by microorganisms. ASDC *J Dent Child.* 56: 201-4.

165. Caudry, S.D., A Klitorinos and EC Chan. 1995. Contaminated toothbrushes and their disinfection. *J Can Dent Assoc* 61(6): 511-6.

166. Glass, R.T. and H.G. Jensen. 1994. The effectiveness of a u-v toothbrush sanitizing device in reducing the number of bacteria, yeasts and viruses on toothbrushes. *J Okla Dent Assoc* 84(4):24-8.

167. Glass, R.T. and H.G. Jensen. 1988. More on the contaminated toothbrush: the viral story. *Quintessence Int* 19:713-6.

168. Warren, D.P. et al. 2001. The effects of toothpastes on the residual microbial contamination of toothbrushes. *JADA* 132:1241-5.

169. Yukna, R.A. et al. 1993. Interproximal vs midradicular effects of a counter-rotational powered brush during supportive periodontal therapy. *Compendium* 16: S580-6.

170. Yuka, R.A. et al. 1993. Evaluation of counter-rotational powered brush in patients in supportive periodontal therapy. *J Periodontal* 64:859-64.

171. Stanford, C.M. et al. 1997. Efficacy of the Sonicare toothbrush fluid dynamic action on removal of human supraginigival plaque. *J Clin Dent.* Special issue: 10-4.

172. Otomo-Corgel, J. 1992. Over-the-counter and prescription mouthwashes - an update for the 1990's. *Compendium of Continuing Dental Education in Dentistry* 13:1086-1095.

173. Lamberts, D.M. et al. 1982. The effect of waxed and unwaxed dental floss on gingival response. *J Periodontol* 53: 393-6.

174. Wunderlich, R.C. et al. 1982. The effect of waxed and unwaxed dental floss on gingival response. *J Periodontol.* 53: 397-400.

175. Gross, A. et al. 1975. Effects of tongue brushing on tongue coating and dental plaque scores. *J Dent Res.* 54:1236.

176. Christen, A.G. et al. 1978. Oral hygiene: a history of tongue scraping and brushing. *JADA* 96: 215-9.

177. Wunderlick, R.C. et al. 1984. Subgingival penetration of an applied solution. *Int J Perio Restorative Dent.* 4 (5): 64-71.

178. Waerhaug, J. 1981. Effect of tooth brushing on subgingival plaque formation. *J Periodontol.* 52(1): 30-4.

179. The role of supra and subgingival irrigation in the treatment of periodontal diseases. 1996. *Chicago: American Academy of Periodontics* 1-18.

180. Eakle, W.S., C. Ford and R.L. Boyd. 1986. Depth of penetration in periodontal pockets with oral irrigation. *J Clin Periodontal* 13(1): 39-44.

181. Larner, J.R. and G. Greenstein. 1993. Effect of calculus and irrigation tip design on depth of subgingival irrigation. *Int. J Periodontics Restorative Dent.* 13(3): 288-97.

182. Braun, R.E. and S.G. Chancio. 1992. Subgingival delivery by an oral irrigation device. *J Periodontal.* 63: 469-72.

183.Newman, et al. 1994. Effectiveness of Adjunctive Irrigation in Early Periodontitis: Multi-Center Evaluation. *J Periodontal* 65:224-229.

184. Nelson, S. 2000. Sodium bicarbonate inhibits plaque formation on teeth. *Dentist.* 68: 23-38.

185. Legier-Vargas, et al. 1995. Effects of sodium bicarbonate dentifrices on the levels of bacteria in human saliva. *Caries Res.* 29: 143-147.

186. Tanzer, et al. Bicarbonate-based powder and paste dentifrice effects on caries. *Clin Prev Den.* 12: 18-21.

187. Koertge, et al. 1998. Longitudinal comparison of tooth whitening resulting from dentifrice use. *J Clin Dent.* 9:67-71.

188. Ody, P. 2000. *Natural Health, Complete Guide to Medicinal Herbs.* New York: Darling Kindersley.

189. Graedon, et al. 1999. *The People's Pharmacy Guide to Home and Herbal Remedies.* New York: St. Martin's Griffin.

190. Hildebrandt, G.H. and B.S. Sparks. 2000. Maintaining *mutans streptococci* suppression with xylitol chewing gum. *J Am Dent Assoc.* 131: 909-916.

191. Vogel, et al. 1978. The effect of folic acid on gingival health, *J Periodontol* 47(11): 667-668.

192. Caranza, F. 1984. *Clinical Periodontology.* Philadelphia: WB Saunders.

193. Sinatra, S. 1999. *L-Carnitine and the Heart, How the powerful combination of L-caritine and CoQ10 can have a positive impact on one's health and well-being.* Los Angeles: Keats Publishing.

194. Weyers, W. et al. 1989.Skin absorption of volatile oils. *Pharmacokinetics Pharm Unsrer Seit* 18: (3):82-6.

195. Packer, L. 2000. *Alpha Lipoic Acid as a biological antioxidant*, Free Radical Biology and Medicine.

196. da Costa, et al. 1974. Appearance of folate binder in leukocytes and serum of women who are pregnant or taking oral contraceptives. *J Lab Clin Med* 83:207-214.

197. Vogel, et al. 1976. The effect of folic acid on gingival health. *J Periodontol* 47(11):667-668.

198. Vogel, et al. 1979. The effect of topical application of folic acid on gingival health. *J Oral Med* 33 (1):20-2.

199. Thompson, et al. 1982. Effects of extended systemic and topical folate supplementation on gingivitis of pregnancy. *J Clin Periodontol* ((9):275-80.

200. Pack, et al. 1980. Effects of topical and systemic folic acid supplementation on gingivitis in pregnancy. *J Clin Periodontol* 7(5): 402-414.

201. Pack, et al. 1984. Folate mouthwash: effects on established gingivitis in periodontal patients. *J Clin Periodontol* 11(9) :619-628.

202. Vogel, et al. 1976. The effect of folic acid on gingival health. *J Periodontol* 47(11):667-668.

203. Adhikari, et al. 2001. Free radical scavenging behavior of folic acid: Evidence for possible antioxidant activity. *Free Radical Biology & Medicine.* 30 (12): 1390-1399.

204. Cohen, et al. 1986. Safety of pyridoxine-A review of human and animal studies. *Toxicol Letters* 34: 129-139.

205.Mason, et al. 1992. The effects of vitamins B12, B6 and folate on blood homocysteine levels. *Ann NY Acad Sci.* 669:197-203.

206. Lubec, et al. 1996. Evidence for McKusick's hypothesis of deficient collagen cross-linking in patients with homocysteine. *Biochim Biophys Acta* 1315(3):159-162.

207. Brattstrom, et al. 1985. Folic acid responsive postmenopausal homocysteinemia. *Metabolism* 34 (11): 1073-1077.

208. Wilcken, et al. 1985. Homocystinuria due to cystathionine beta-synthase deficiency-the effects of betaine treatment in pyridoxine-responsive patients, *Metabolism* 34 (12):115-1121.

209. Dorman, H. 2000. Antimicrobial agents from plants: Antibacterial activity of plant volatile oils. *J of Applied Microbiology* 88 (2): 308-316.

210. Badmaev, et al. 1996. *Comparison of nutrient bioavailability when ingested alone and in combination with Bioperine, Research Report,* Sabinsa Corporation.

211. Ibid.

212. Clark, H. 1993. The Cure for All Cancers. San Dieo: ProMotion Publishing.

213. Godowski, K.C. 1989. Antimicrobial action of sanguinarine. *J Clin Dent* 1: 96-101.

214. Nielson, F.H. 1990. Studies on the relationship between boron and magnesium, which possibly effect the formation and maintenance of bones. *Magnesium Trace Elem* 9:61-69.

215. Frei, et al. 1989. Ascorbate is an outstanding antioxidant in human blood plasma. *Proc Natl Acad Sci* 86: 66377-81.

216. Nakamoto, et al. The role of ascorbic acid deficiency in human gingivitis-a new hypothesis. *J Theor Biol* 108 (2):163-171.

217. Goetzl, et al. 1974. Enhancement of random migration and chemotactic response of human leukocytes by ascorbic acid. *J Clin Invest* 53 : 813.

218. Thomas, et al. 1978. Vitamin C and immunity: an assessment of the evidence. *Clin Exptl Immunol* 32: 370.

219. Rivers, J.M. 1989. Safety of high level vitamin C ingestion. *Int J Vit Ntr Res* 30 (Suppl): 95-102.

220. Abraham, et al. 1990. Total dietary program emphasizing magnesium instead of calcium. *J Repro Med* 35 (5): 503-507.

221. Abraham, G.E. 1982. The calcium controversy. *J Appl Nutr* 34: 69.

222. Bourgoin, et al. 1993. Lead Content in 70 Brands of Dietary Calcium Supplements. *Am J Public Health* 83 :1155-60.

223. Hoffman, D. 1983. *The Holistic Herbal.* Scotland: Findhorn Press.

224. Haines, C.E. 1994. Antimutagenesis and Lethality Studies of Cinnamaldehyde in Bacterial Systems. *University of Kansas* 56 (04B).

225. Tantaoui-Elaraki, et al. 1994. Inhibition of growth and aflatoxin production in Aspergillus parasiticus by essential oils of selected plant materials. *J Environ Pathol Toxicol Oncol* 13 (1):67-72.

226. Goldenberg, R. 1997. Drug and Cosmetic Industry. 06.

227. Inouye, et al. 1998. Antisporulating and respiration-inhibitory effects of essential oils on filamentous fungi. *Mycose* 41 (9-10): 403-10.

228. Jayashree, et al. 1999. Anti-aflatoxigenic activity of eugenol is due to inhibition of lipid peroxidation. *Lett Appl Microbiol.* 28(3):179-83.

229. Wie, et al. 1997. Eugenol protects neuronal cells from excitotoxic and oxidative injury in primary cortical cultures. *Neurosci Lett,* 4 ;225(2):93-96.

230. Siddiqui, et al. 1996. Effect of essential oils on the enveloped viruses : Antiviral activity of oregano and clove oils on herpes simplex virus type 1 and Newcastle disease virus. *Medical Science Research* 24 (3):185-186.

231. Hansen, et al. 1976. Bioenergetics in clinical therapy. Gingival and leucocytic deficiencies of coenzyme Q10 in patients with periodontal disease. *Res Commun Chem Pathol Pharmacol* 14(4): 729-738.

232. Matsumura, et al. 1973. Evidence for enhanced treatment of periodontal disease by therapy with coenzyme Q. *Int J Vitam Nutr Res* 43 (4):537-548.

233. Nakamura, et al. 1974. Study of coenzyme Q in gingival of patients with periodontal disease and evidence for a deficiency of coenzyme Q10. *Proc Natt Acad Sci* 71:1456.

234. Batino, et al. 1999. Oxidative injury and inflammatory diseases: the challenge of antioxidants to free radicals and reactive oxygen speies. *Crit Rev Oral Biol Med* 10(4): 458-76.

235. Folkers, et al. 1981. *Biomedical and Clinical Aspects of Coenzyme Q.* vol. 3, Amsterdam: Elsevier/North Holland Biomedical Press.

236. Wilkinson, et al. 1977. *Treatment of periodontal and other soft tissue diseases of the oral cavity with coenzyme Q. In Biomedical and Clinical Aspects of Coenzyme Q administration.* Vol. 1 Folkers K and Yamamura Y (eds.) Elsevier/North-Hollarn Biomedical Press, Amsterdam.

237. Hanioka, et al. 1994. Effect of topical application of coenzyme Q10 on adult Periodontitis. *Mol Aspects Med* 15 Suppl: 241-248.

238. Emile, et al. 1987. *The Miracle Nutrient CoEnzymeQ10.* New York: Bantam Books.

239. Lewis, A.J. 1984. The role of Copper in Inflammatory Disorders. *Agents Actions.*

240. Airola, P. 1976. *How to Get Well. Health.* Phoenix: Plus Publishers.

241. Kim, et al. 1983. The effect of Vitamin E on the Healing of Gingival Wounds in rats. *J Periodontal* 54:305-8.

242. Royack, et al. 2000. Response of human oral epithelial cells to oxidative damage and the effect of vitamin E. *Oral Oncology* 36(1):37-41.

243. Addya, et al. 1984. Effects of Mercuric Chloride on Several Scavenging Enzymes in Rat Kidney and Influence of Vitamin E Supplementation. *Acta Vitaminol Encymol* 6;103-107.

244. Courtney, et al. 1991. Aggregation of group A streptococci by human saliva and effect of saliva on streptococcal adherence to host cells. *Infect Immun.* 59(5): 1661-1666.

245. D'Amelio, F. 1999. *Botanicals, A Phytocosmetic Desk Reference.* Boca Raton: CRC Press.

246. Wagner, et al. 1989. In vitro inhibition of arachidonate *metabolism* by some alkylamides and phenylated phenols. *Planta Medica.* 55:566-567.

247. Wagner, et al. 1985. Immunostimulating polysaccharides (heteroglycans) of higher plants. *Arzneimittel-Forsch* 35: 1069-75.

248. Hobbs, C. 1989. *The Echinacea Handbook.* Portland: Eclectic Medical Publications.

249. Bauer, et al. 1991. Echinacea species as potential immunostimulatory drugs. *Econ Med Plant Res* 5: 253-321.

250. D'Amelio, F. 1999. *Botanicals, A Phytocosmetic Desk Reference.* Boca Raton: CRC Press.

251. Weyer, et al. 1989. Skin absorption of volatile oils. Pharmacoinetics. *Pharm Unsrer Seit* 18 (3): 82-86.

252. D'Amelio, F. 1999. *Botanicals, A Phytocosmetic Desk Reference.* Boca Raton: CRC Press.

253. Boiteau, et al. 1956. Asiaticoside. Extracted from Centella asistica. Its therapeutic uses in the healing of experimental or refractory wounds, leprosy, skin tuberculosis and lupus. *Therapie* 11: 125-149.

254. Tenni, et al. 1988. Effect of the triterpenoid fraction of Centella Asiatica: on macromolecules of the connective matrix in human skin fibroblast cultures. *Ital J Biochem* 37:69-77.

255. Shukla, et al. 1999. Asiaticoside induced elevation of antioxidant levels in healing wounds *Phytother Res* 13:50-54.

256. Suguna, L. 1996. Effects of Centella asiatica extract on dermal wound healing in rats. *Indian J Exp Biol* 34 (12):1208-11.

257. Antibiotic Alternative Proven Effective, The GSE Report 1:1, 1.

258. Masquelier, J. 1990. Procyanidolic oligomers. *J Parfums Cosmet Arom.* 95:89-97.

259. Laparra, J. 1978. Parmacokinetic study of the total procyanidolic oligomers of the grape. *Acta Therapeutica.* 4: 233-246.

260. Hagerman, et al. 1981. The specificity of Proanthocyanidin-Protein interactions. *Journ of Biol Chemistry* 256: 4494-4497.

261. Sorsa, et al. 1990. The role of gingival crevicular fluid and salivary interstitial collagenases in human periodontal diseases. *Arch Oral Biol Supp.* 35: 193-196.

262. Nakamura, M. 1979. The relationship between periodontal disease and protease activity in gingival fluid and in saliva. *Nippon Shishubyo Gakkai Kaishi.* 21(4): 429-434.

263. Inoue, J. 1990. Distribution of enzymatically pathogenic bacteria from periodontal pocket in advancing periodontitis. *Nippon Shishubyo Gakkai Kaishi.* 32(1): 199-205.

264. Bombardelli, et al. 1996. Aesculus hipposcastanu. *Fitoterapia* Vol LXVII (6): 503.

265. Gilman, et al. 1980. The Pharmacological Basis of Therapeutics, 6th edition.

266. Reimann, et al. 1977. Histamine and acute haemorrhagic lesions in rat gastric mucosa: prevention of stress ulcer formation by (+)- catechin, an inhibitor of specific histidine decarboxylase in vitro. *Agents Actions* 7(1): 69-73.

267. Amelia, et al. 1985. Inhibition of mast cell histamine release by flavonoids and bioflavonoids. *Planta Medica* 5116-20.

268. Uchida, et al. 1987. Condensed tannins scavage active oxygen radicals. *Med Sci Res.* 15: 831-832.

269. Montogomery, et al. 1993. *Biochemistry.* 4th edition. St. Louis: Mosby Company.

270. Price, PA. 1993. Vitamin K nutrition and postmenopausal osteoporosis. *J Clin Invest* 91(4):1268.

271. Lorrondo, et al. 1995. Antimicrobial activity of essences from labiates. *Microbios* 82 (332): 171-2.

272. Combest, WL. 1999. Lavender. *US Pharmacist* (USA) 24: 30-33.

273. Petrovski, S. 1888. Study of the antibacterial and antimycotic action of lavender essential oil. *Dermatol Veneral.* 27 (3):46-50.

274. Perrucci, et al. 1994. Acaricidal agents of natural origin against Psoroptes cuniculi. *Parassitologia* 36(3): 269-271.

275. Nelson, R. 1997. In-vitro activities of five plant essential oils against methicillin-resistant Staphylococcus aureus and vancomycin-resistant Enterococcu faecium. *Journal of Antimicrobial Chemotherapy* 40 (2): 305-306.

276. Almer, et al. 1992. Pharmacokinetics of tranexamic acid in patients with ulcerative colitis and in healthy volunteers after the single instillation of 2 g rectally. *Journal of Clinical Pharmacology* 32: 49-54.

277. Astedt, et al. 1977. Arrest of growth of ovarian tumour by ranexamic acid. *Journal of the American Medical Assoc.* 238: 154-155.

278. Rath, M. 1992. Plasmin induced proteolysis and the role of apoprotein(a), lysine and synthetic lysine analogs. *Journal of Orthomolecular Medicine* 7:17-23.

279. Rath, M. 2001. *Cellular Health Series: The Heart.* Santa Clara, Calif. MR Publishing, Inc.

280. Sigurdsson, et al. Tranexamic acid for the treatment of advanced ovarian carcinoma. *Acta Obstetriticia et Gynecologica Scandinavica* 62: 265-266.

281. Balch, P., and J. Balch. 2000. *Prescription for Nutritional Healing.* New York: Penguin Putnam, Inc.

282. Birkmayer, J.G.D., Biological and Clinical Relevance of Trace Elements. *Arztl Lab* 36: 284-87, 1990.

283. Balch, et al. 2000. *Prescription for Nutritional Healing,* 3rd ed. New York: Avery Publishing.

284. Tranter, H.S. 1993. The effect of the olive phenolic compound, oleuropein, on growth and enterotoxin B production by Staphylococcus aureus. *Journal of Applied Bacteriology* 74 (3): 253-259.

285. Fleming, H.P. 1973. Antimicrobial properties of oleuropein and products of its hydrolysis from green olives. *Applied Microbiology* 26 (5): 777-782.

286. Petkov, et al. 1972. Pharmacological analysis of iridoid oleuropein. *Drug Res.* 22 (9): 1476-86.

287. Walker, M. 1997. *Nature's Antibiotic Olive Leaf Extract,* Kensington Books, Kensington Publishing Corp.

288. Tassou, C. 1991. Effect of phenolic compounds and oleuropein on the germination of Bacullus cereus T spores. *Biotechnology and Applied Biochemistry* 13:231-237.

289. Stiles, et al. 1995. The inhibition of Candida Albicans by oregano. *J Applied Nutr* 47: 96-102.

290. Draughon, et al. 2001. Antimicrobial activity of essential oils from plants against selected pathogenic and saprophytic microorganisms. *Journal of Food Protection* 42 (7): 1019-24.

291. Baratta, M.T. 1998. Chemical composition, antimicrobial and antioxidative activity of laurel, sage. Rosemary, oregano and coriander essential oils. *Journal of Essential Oil Research* 10 (6): 618-627.

292. Sivropoulou, A. 1996. Antimicrobial and cytotoxic activities of Origanum essential oils. *J. Agric Food Chem.* 5: 1202-1205.

293. Kivanc, M. Inhibitory and stimulatory effects of cumin, oregano and their essential oils on growth and acid production of Lactobacillus plantarum.

294. Daouk, et al. 1995. Antifungal activity of the essential oil of Origanum syriacum L. *Journal of Food Protection* 58 (10).

295. Siddiqui, et al. 1996. Effect of essential oils on the enveloped viruses : Antiviral activity of oregano and clove oils on herpes simplex virus type 1 and Newcastle disease virus. *Medical Science Research* 24 (3): 185-186.

296. Hammer, et al. 1999. Antimicrobial activity of essential oils and other plant extracts. *Journal of Applied Microbiology* 86 (6): 985-990.

297. Samman, et al. 1998. Mint prevents carcinogenesis in hamster cheek pouch. 19 (10): 1795-801.

298. May, et al. 1996. Efficacy of a fixed peppermint oil/caraway oil combination in non-ulcer dyspepsia. *Arzneim Forsch* 46:1149-53.

299. Hassanein, et al. 1997. Antibacterial action of carvone and some plant extracts on certain phytopathogenic bacteria and pathogenicity of Agro bacterium tumefaciens. *Alexandria Journal of Agricultural Research* 42 (1): 127-136.

300. Yu, et al. 1994. *Phytotherapy Res.* 8(7): 436.

301. Lee, et al. 1988. *Mutat Res.* 204 (2): 229.

302. Lin, et al. 1973. *Microbiol.* 6: 97.

303. Jacobs, et al. U.S. Patent No. 4,745,104 (May 17,1988 and No. 4, 849,410 (July 18,1989).

304. Howell, E. 1985. *Enzyme Nutrition.* Wayne, New Jersey: Avery Publishing Group.

305. Hoffman, D. 1983. *The Holistic Herbal.* Scotland: Findhorn Press..

306. Rath, M. 2001. *Cellular Health Series: Cancer.* California: MR Publishing.

307. Pearce, et al. 1984. Mucosal Mast Cells III: Effect of Quercetin and Other Flavonoids on Antigen-Induced Histamine Secretion from Rat Intestinal Mast Cells. *J Allergy Clin Immunol* 73:819-23.

308. Busse, et al. 1984. Flavonoid Modulation of Human Neutrophil Function. *J Allergy Clin Immunol* 73: 801-9.

309. Yoshimoto, T. 1983. Flavonoids: Potent inhibitors of Archidonate 5-Lipoxygenase. *Biochem Biophys Res Comm.* 116:612-18.

310. D'Amelio, F. 1999. *Botanicals, A Phytocosmetic Desk Reference.* Boca Raton: CRC Press.

311. Roy, M. 1994. Supplementation with Selenium and Human Imune Cell Functions II: Effect on Lymphocytes Proliferation and Interleudin 2 Receptor Expression. *Biol Trace Elem Res.* 41:103-14.

312. Kiremidjian-Schumacher, et al. 1994. Supplementation with Selenium and Human Immune Cell Functions II: Effect on Cytotoxic Lymphocytes and Natural Killer Cells. *Biol Trace Elem Res.* 41:115-27.

313. Carlisle, E.M. 1982. The Nutritional Essentiality of Silicon. *Nutr Rev* 40 (7): 193-198.

314. Fessenden, et al. 1987. The Biological Properties of Silicon Compounds. *Adv Drug Res.* 4:95.

315. Ultee, et al. 1999. Bactericidal activity of carvacrol towards the food-borne pathogen Bacillus cereus. 85 (2): 211-218.

316. Lisin, et al. 1999. Antimicrobial activity of some essential oils. *Acta Horticulrurae* (501): 283-288.

317. Marino, et al. 1999. Antimicrobial activity of the essential oils of Thymus vulgaris L. measured using a bioimpedometric method. *J Food Prot.* 62 (9): 1017-23.

318. Juven, et al. 1994. Factors that interact with the antibacterial action of thyme essential oil and its active constituents. *J Appl Bacteriol* 76 (6):626-31.

319. Tzakou, et al. 1998. Chemical composition and antibacterial properties of Thymus longicaulis subsp.chaoubardii oils: three chemotypes in the same population. *Journal of Essential Oil Research* 10 (1): 97-99.

320. Hassanein, et al. 1997. Antibacterial action of carvone and some plant extracts on certain phytopathogenic bacteria and pathogenicity of Agrobacterium tumefaciens. *Alexandria Journal of Agricultural Research.* 42 (1): 127-136.

321. Lattaoui, et al. 1994. Comparative kinetics of microbial destruction by the essential oils of Thymus broussonettii, T. zygis and T. satureioides. *Journal of Essential Oil Research* 6 (2): 106-171.

322. Panizzi, et al. 1993. Composition and antimicrobial properties of essential oils of four Mediterranean Lamiaceae. *J Ethnopharmacol.* 39 (3): 167-70.

323. Hildebrandt, et al. 2000. Maintaining *mutans streptococci* suppression with xylitol chewing gum. *J Am Dent Assoc.* 131: 909-916.

324. Prasad, A. 1983. Clinical Biochemical and Nutritional Spectrum of Zinc Deficiency in Human Subjects: An Update. *Nutr Rev.* 41: 197-208.

325. Freeland, et al. 1976. Relationship of Mineral Status and Intake to Periodontal Disease. *Am J Clin Nutr.* 29: 745-9

Index

Give the gift of great oral health!

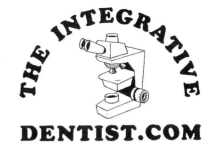

YES, I want _____ copies of *The Periodontal Solution: Healthy Gums Naturally* at $14.95 each $_____

Add $5.00 shipping and handling for 1st copy; $1.50 for additional copies   _____

Florida residents, add 6% sales tax   _____

    Total $_____

My check or money order for $_____, payable to Corinthian Health Press, is enclosed.

Please charge my   VISA   MasterCard

Card number: _____

Expiration date (mm/yy): _____

Cardholder's signature: _____

Shipping Information

Name _____

Address _____

City/State/Zip _____

Phone _____ E-mail _____

Send completed order form to:

Corinthian Health Press
1730 Federal Highway, Suite 206
Delray Beach, FL 33483

Or order by:

Phone: 561/704-0038
E-mail: orders@theintegrativedentist.com

Notes

Notes

Notes

About the Author

ollowing his graduation from the University of Vermont in Engineering, James Harrison, D.D.S. received his dental training at the State University of New York at Buffalo. After graduation, he joined the faculty in fixed prosthetics for two years.

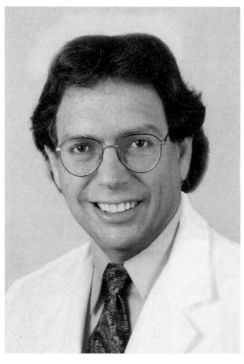

He is a fellow and a director of the International Academy of Oral Medicine and Toxicology. He is a fellow of the Academy of General Dentistry and a member of the Academy of Cosmetic Dentistry, the Environmental Medical Association, the Holistic Dental Association and the American Dental Association. In addition he has experienced and studied healing systems around the world. In his private practice in Lake Worth, Florida, he specializes in integrative dentistry.

Dr. Harrison can be reached through his website, *theintegrativedentist.com* or e-mail at *dr.jim@harrison.net*. He is also available for private phone consultations at 561-626-9879.